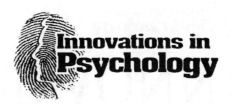

BURNOUT
in FAMILIES
The Systemic Costs of Caring

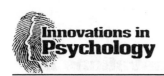

INNOVATIONS
in PSYCHOLOGY

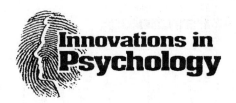

BURNOUT

in FAMILIES

The Systemic Costs of Caring

Edited by
Charles R. Figley, Ph.D.

CRC Press

Boca Raton   Boston   New York   Washington   London

Library of Congress Cataloging-in-Publication Data

Catalog record is available from the Library of Congress.

This book contains information obtained from authentic and highly regarded sources. Reprinted material is quoted with permission, and sources are indicated. A wide variety of references are listed. Reasonable efforts have been made to publish reliable data and information, but the author and the publisher cannot assume responsibility for the validity of all materials or for the consequences of their use.

Neither this book nor any part may be reproduced or transmitted in any form or by any means, electronic or mechanical, including photocopying, microfilming, and recording, or by any information storage or retrieval system, without prior permission in writing from the publisher.

All rights reserved. Authorization to photocopy items for internal or personal use, or the personal or internal use of specific clients, may be granted by CRC Press LLC, provided that $.50 per page photocopied is paid directly to Copyright Clearance Center, 27 Congress Street, Salem, MA 01970 USA. The fee code for users of the Transactional Reporting Service is ISBN 0-57444-047-0/97/ $0.00+$.50. The fee is subject to change without notice. For organizations that have been granted a photocopy license by the CCC, a separate system of payment has been arranged.

The consent of CRC Press LLC does not extend to copying for general distribution, for promotion, for creating new works, or for resale. Specific permission must be obtained in writing from CRC Press LLC for such copying.

Direct all inquiries to CRC Press LLC, 2000 Corporate Blvd., N.W., Boca Raton, Florida 33431.

Trademark Notice: Product or corporate names may be trademarks or registered trademarks, and are used only for identification and explanation, without intent to infringe.

© 1998 by CRC Press LLC

No claim to original U.S. Government works
International Standard Book Number 0-57444-047-0
Printed in the United States of America 1 2 3 4 5 6 7 8 9 0

EDITORIAL NOTE BY THE SERIES EDITOR

This is the first in this Book Series, *Innovations in Psychology*. The Series was established in 1996 to stimulate the field of psychology. As a long-time Fellow of the American Psychological Association, I have always stimulated innovation among my students and colleagues. I have also made a few contributions myself along the way.

The purpose of this Book Series is to publish books that contribute to psychology through the explication of creative changes in the way we view various phenomenon that can be studied and treated by psychologists. This is not to say that the applications do not go far beyond psychology. This first book, for example, should make useful contributions to family therapy, social work, traumatology, and other fields in addition to psychology.

A large percentage of the books to be published in this Series, however, will be limited to psychologists. Similarly, the distinguished list of psychologists on our Editorial Board include several well-known psychologists with others joining shortly. However, there are physicians, social workers, family therapists, and others on the Board who, together, are in an excellent position of judging the quality of book proposals as innovations in psychology.

In this volume, *Burnout in Families*, the innovation is applying the concepts, measures, theories, and treatments that appear to be useful in the work setting to family settings. Moreover, the understanding of couples, marriages, parent–child, and sibling–sibling relationships. Reframing marital breakdown as burnout, for example, provides a more optimistic view for preventing divorce and treating the underlying problems that lead to this outcome.

This book evolved from a research project focusing on compassion fatigue, a form of burnout, among psychologists and others who study and treat suffering clients. This is the second book to emerge from that study. The first book, *Compassion Fatigue* (Figley, 1995) received critical acclaim (e.g., Mitchell, 1996). Given the quality of the contributors and the importance of the topic, we expect that this volume will receive similar, positive attention.

If you are interested in the Series considering your book or those of your colleagues, please write us via the St. Lucie Publishing Group at CRC Press LLC.

The publisher, Editorial Board, and I look forward to your reactions and recommendations.

Charles R. Figley, Ph.D.
Professor and Series Editor

CONTRIBUTING AUTHORS

Michael F. Barnes, Ph.D.
Director
Residential Treatment Facility
Charter Behavioral Health
  System at Cove Forge
Williamsburg, Pennsylvania

Donald R. Catherall, Ph.D.
Executive Director
The Phoenix Institute
Chicago, Ilinois

Robert A. Ferguson, Ph.D.
Counseling and Testing Center
University of Kentucky
Lexington, Kentucky

Charles R. Figley, Ph.D.
Interdivisional Ph.D. Program
  in Marriage and Family
Florida State University
Tallahassee, Florida

Kathleen Gilbert, Ph.D.
Associate Professor
Department of Applied Health
  Science
Indiana University
Bloomington, Indiana

Rory Remer, Ph.D.
Professor and Director of
  Graduate Studies
Department of Educational and
  Counseling Psychology
University of Kentucky
Lexington, Kentucky

Arlene Steinberg, Psy.D.
Adjunct Assistant Professor
Teacher's College Columbia
  University
Private Practice
New York, New York

Mary Beth Williams, Ph.D.
Director
Institute for Traumatized
  Children
Warringtonn, Virginia

TABLE OF CONTENTS

INTRODUCTION

Charles R. Figley, Ph.D.

Conceptually, the term "burnout" in families may seem odd. After all, the dictionary definition of burnout is a noun meaning "termination of the powered portion of a rocket's flight upon exhaustion of the propellant" (*Random House Dictionary*). Thus, burnout in families might be considered a sign of family members running out of gas.

This book is a collection of chapters that observe how families experience and cope with psychosocial stress or experience various forms of burnout when they fail to cope. Here, we intend to introduce the reader to some of the critical concepts used throughout this book, starting with burnout, and ways of thinking about these concepts that will be useful in reading and applying the coming chapters to the reader's own work with individuals and families who wish to improve the overall quality of family life.

Burnout was introduced to the scientific literature in 1974 by Herbert J. Freudenberger (1974) in his classic article, "Staff Burnout," published in the *Journal of Social Issues*. Shortly thereafter, Christina Maslach (1976), a social psychologist, published the first in a series of studies to share and refine the meaning and measurement of the concept. Recently, Pines (1993) noted that a *Psychological Abstracts* search revealed more than 1000 research articles and close to 100 books on burnout.

Pines & Aronson (1988) define burnout as a "...state of physical, emotional, and mental exhaustion caused by long term involvement in emotionally demanding situations" (p. 9). Most often burnout has been associated with an accumulation of stressors that erode the individual's high ideals, motivations, and commitments to a particular field, profession, career, or job.

1-57444-047-0/98/$0.00+$.50
© 1998 by CRC Press LLC

1

In this book, we apply this construct to family life ideals, motivations to remain in the family, and commitments to the family as evidenced by expressions of love, and to actions that further and support the family and its members. Of most concern in this collection is the impact of highly stressful events that are often imposed on the family through one of its members. Chapter 1 fully explores the conceptual and clinical implications of burnout in families. Some of the more basic concepts are noted here, following a discussion of the way family crisis and stress have been viewed in the literature.

MODELS OF FAMILY STRESS AND CRISIS

Reuben (1949), in his classic study of family stress of returning World War II veterans' families, first suggested how families deal with crisis and applied the newly coined concept of stress. Also, he was the first to suggest that the system of the family is greatly affected by crisis events such as war and post-war reunion. Most agree that Hill origi-nated the concept of family stress (Figley, 1989). This sociological orientation emerged into what was later called the ABCX Model (Hill & Hansen, 1965) and most recently articulated by McCubbin and McCubbin (1989) as their Typology Model of Family Adjustment and Adaptation. They suggest that the family's adjustment to a stressor is mediated by what they describe as family vulnerability (V Factor), defined as the interpersonal and organizational condition of the family system shaped, in part, by (a) a pileup of demands on the family and (b) the family's life-cycle stage-related stressors and access to methods of coping (Olson et al., 1983). This, in turn, is mediated by the type of family function (T Factor), which is defined as a set of basic attributes about the family system which characterizes and explains how a family system typically appraises, operates, and/or behaves. For example, Balanced Families (Lavee, 1985) respond more supportively and with greater ease to stressors and appear to be more resistant to negative health outcomes. Regenerative Families (McCubbin, Thompson, Pirner & McCubbin, 1988) are better able to manage hardships and promote other family strengths of bonding, flexibility, and predictability, as well as marital and family satisfaction.

Alternatively, one could simply measure the degree of stress resis-tance or resiliency in the family rather than using statistically limiting categorical concepts such as the T Factor. The B Factor in the McCubbin and McCubbin (1989) model is resistance resources or the ability of the family to recognize, plan, and implement a method of coping until the stressor is eliminated or effectively resolved. The PSC Factor, family management through problem solving and coping, includes the family's strategies, patterns, and behaviors designated to (1) maintain and/or strengthen the organization and stability of the family unit, (2) maintain the emotional stability and well-being of the family members, (3) obtain and/or utilize family and community resources to manage the situation, and (4) initiate efforts to resolve the family hardships created by the stressor (McCubbin & McCubbin, 1989, p. 10).

A new model of secondary traumatic stress disorder and family burnout is discussed in Chapter 1. It incorporates the latter three factors, T, B, and PSC Factors, to form a single –A– Factor. The A Factor represents the general level of adaptability, a general measure of the overall flexibility, resiliency, and morale within the family, suggesting the degree to which each family member is willing to change and adapt to cope with the stressor as a family. This is an ongoing process of attempting to solve problems by solutions that at least do no harm to the family and preferably make it stronger and better able to cope with future adversities based on what family members have learned.

Modern family stress specialists also suggest that there is an X Factor in family stress reactions — the resultant stress and distress within the family, in spite of or perhaps because of the family's initial efforts to cope. Some call this a state of crisis (McCubbin & McCubbin, 1989) but it could be conceived as a state of distress or high stress that requires immediate attention to reduce before there is burnout — either temporary or permanent.

Family crisis has been conceptualized as a continuous variable denoting the amount of disruptiveness, disorganization, or incapacitation in the family social system (Burr, 1973). Crisis is a state of family system disorganization, whereas family stress is a state of tension brought about by the demand–capability imbalance in the family. It is as if crisis occurs when family stress reaches a critically high level. Although the crisis state is transitional, families that must endure this state for very long are highly vulnerable to family burnout and its consequences, including family violence, and violations of the family standards and norms (e.g., cheating).

McCubbin and McCubbin (1989) also suggest that there is a family adaptation phase, which is the mirror response to the family adjustment phase. The adaptation phase of their Typology Model of Adjustment and Adaptation suggests that family adaptation to crisis and more chronic stressors is a function of eight factors:

1. Current (pileup of) demands (AA Factor)
   which influences
2. Utilization of family resources (R Factor)
   which influences
3. The T Factor (the type of family as a function of the degree of family coherence and hardiness)
   which influences both
4. The CC Factor (family appraisal), which is influenced by the CCC Factor (global appraisal or the family schema)
5. The BB Factor (the family's resistance capabilities and stratagems of coping)
   which is influenced by
6. The BBB Factor (community resources and supports)
7. The PSC Factor (indices of effective family management)
   which is directly related to
8. The XX Factor (the overall adaptability of the family to cope with the crisis)

Perhaps more importantly, McCubbin and McCubbin (1989) predict from this model eight types of families based on the degree to which the family is either high or low in family bonding, family flexibility, family coherence, and family hardiness. The first type, *Vulnerable Families* (low coherence and low hardiness), requires the most attention from service providers. *Regenerative Families* (high coherence and high hardiness) require the least attention. *Durable Families,* although high in coherence, are low in hardiness. *Secure Families* are high in hardiness but low in coherence. At the same time, the authors suggest that *Resilient Families* are those with both high family bonding and high family flexibility. *Fragile Families* are those with both low family bonding and low family flexibility. *Pliant Families* are high in flexibility but low in bonding, whereas *Bonded Families* are high in bonding but low in flexibility. They suggest that each of these families varies in the extent to which it is able to solve the problems caused by recent or ongoing stressor challenges demanding action.

In terms of burnout, the families at greatest risk are the *Fragile Families*, as indicated by low family bonding and flexibility. They are "...hesitant to depend upon the family for support and understanding, prefer to confide in persons outside the family, avoid other family members, have difficulty in doing things with the family, and feel that the family emphasizes members going their own way. Additionally, these families perceive themselves as closed in their communication, resistant to compromise, set in their ways and inexperienced in shifting responsibilities among family members, and not involving all family members in making major decisions" (McCubbin & McCubbin, 1989, p. 31).

Vulnerable Families, as indicated by low family coherence and hardiness, appear to handle problems in the family by bursts of emotional reactions, expressing less patience and respect for each another, blaming others, and showing less caring and understanding. They appear to have less pride in and loyalty to their family and less acceptance of family hardships. Additionally, *Vulnerable Families,* compared to other types, indicate a lower sense of purpose, lower meaningfulness in life, and less sense of being appreciated. They appear to feel a sense of helplessness and discouragement. As a result, family members are more prone to stress-related problems such as illness, accidents, and "bad luck" (McCubbin & McCubbin, 1989).

Finally, McCubbin and McCubbin (1989) suggest that the *Unpatterned Families* would also be vulnerable since they do not value and have little experience with family time together and established family routines.

FOCUS OF THE BOOK

Family burnout is defined here as the ultimate fatigue of intimate relationships. Together with my fellow contributors to this book, we focus on the family context affected by a gradual deterioration of the quality and functionality of significant interpersonal relationships. We define family burnout as a family that has suffered fatigue associated with devotion to various family relationships that failed to produce the expected rewards.

Together with my fellow authors, we focus in this book on the family context and how burnout may result when there is a failure of members to work cooperatively to solve various stressful problems. Consistent with Freudenberg's original conceptualization, family burnout is the ultimate fatigue and frustration resulting from a failure to produce expected rewards by family membership.

Of special interest is the concept of secondary stress reactions, including traumatic stress reactions, by family members. These reactions are directly or indirectly caused by the suffering of other family members. The concept of family burnout is useful in characterizing one outcome of these struggles by family members to cope with the suffering of another family member and the impact it has on the family collectively.

Eight family psychologists and systemic traumatologists have collaborated with the editor to produce this book. The book emerged from a larger project focusing on the phenomenon of secondary traumatic stress. The first book from the project focused on the secondary traumatic express experienced by professionals working with the suffering. Because the burnout of such experiences was a direct function of the professionals' compassion and empathy for those clients they serve, the book was titled *Compassion Fatigue: Coping with Secondary Traumatic Stress Disorder in Those Who Treat the Traumatized* (Figley, 1995). As a special form of burnout, compassion fatigue is relevant to family burnout. However, because of the pervasive nature of family life and the complexities of the family system, the concept of burnout seemed best suited to examine and discuss how families cope, or family to cope with stressors members must endure over prolonged periods.

DEFINITIONS OF BASIC CONCEPTS

Families are composed of members who have ongoing and interdependent relationships with one another and one another's outside family and friends. Viewed as a psychosocial system, we are concerned, simultaneously, with the family's structure (arrangement of roles, rules, and expectations for its members) and its processes of acquiring and disseminating social supportiveness and other key resources for its members. A psychosocial system like the family is a living, changing entity of self-correcting and self-sustaining activities that respond to changing demands.

Psychosocial Systemic Stress

Stress, especially in an interpersonal context, is another important concept. Stress, according to Selye (1956, 1974), is a nonspecific (that is, common) result of any demand upon the body, whether the effect is mental or somatic. As he noted most recently, "The formulation of this definition, based on objective indicators such as bodily and chemical changes that appear after any demand, has brought the subject up from the level of cocktail party chitchat into the domain of science" (p. 7). The "demand on the body" in terms of this book is the psychosocial or systemic stressor.

When concentrated doses of stress are introduced into the family, the result is often a systemic or family-wide response that impacts the sources of stress (stressor). Perhaps the most important psychosocial stress is secondary traumatic stress.

Secondary traumatic stress (STS) is the experience of tension and distress directly related to the demands of living with and caring for someone who displays the symptoms of post-traumatic stress disorder (PTSD). STS is associated not only with demands of a family member with PTSD but can also be associated with a feeling of empathy for the traumatic experiences of the loved one.

Secondary traumatic stress disorder (STSD) is the result of a buildup of STS that leads to emotional exhaustion and *emotional burnout,* the focus of this volume. Most of the chapters focus on STSD and provide the basis for an entirely new area of specialization in the fields of both traumatology and family psychology.

Stress leads to burnout both directly and indirectly because it is a solution—giving up and believing those maintaining satisfactory standards of expectations of desired resources. This is when family members often withdraw emotionally or physically or both for various amounts of time. The most drastic impact of burnout in families is ending family ties through abandonment, divorce, or separation, leading to little or no contact.

Systemic traumatology is the study and treatment of groups, institutions, and other human systems exhibiting stress reactions that are a direct result of a traumatic event or series of events

Secondary or systemic traumatic stress is the natural consequent behaviors and emotions resulting from knowledge about a stressful event experienced by a significant other (e.g., family members); it is the stress that results from helping or wanting to help a traumatized person. This concept was first introduced in the early 1980s (cf., Figley, 1982, 1983) and was further articulated by Solomon in a series of studies (cf., Solomon et al., 1987, 1991, 1992).

A *traumatic event* occurs when a person experiences an event outside the range of usual human experience that would be markedly distressing to almost anyone: a serious threat to one's life or physical integrity; serious threat or harm to one's children, spouse, or other close relatives or friends; sudden destruction of one's home or community; or seeing another person seriously injured or killed in an accident or by physical violence (APA, 1994).

Family burnout is the breakdown of the family members' collective commitment to each other and a refusal to work together in harmony as a function of some crisis or traumatic event or series of crises or events that leave members emotionally exhausted and disillusioned.

CONTENT OF THE BOOK

Organizational Structure

In Chapters 1 to 4, the research and practice literature that applies to STS and burnout in families is reviewed. These conceptual chapters address five fundamental questions: (1) What is the family's special context within which systemic traumatic stress is experienced? (2) What are the unintended, and often unexpected, deleterious effects of living with a loved one who is traumatized? (3) What are some examples of those who were indirectly traumatized or burned out as a result of living with a traumatized person? (4) What are the characteristics of the traumatized helper (e.g., race, gender, ethnicity, age, interpersonal competence, experience with psychological trauma) that account for the development, sustenance, preventability, and treatability of secondary traumatization? (5) Is there a way, theoretically, to account for all of these factors?

The other four chapters focus on treatment and prevention: ways of helping, treating, or preventing burnout and other by-products of STS. These chapters address at least one the following questions, building upon the earlier chapters: (1) What are the unique challenges in studying, assessing, and helping families (i.e., helping children, parents, spouses, or the entire family system simultaneously)? (2) What are the characteristics of effective programs to prevent or treat burnout and the unwanted aspects that lead to burnout? (3) What are the implications of the treatment/prevention approach described in this chapter in training a new generation of professionals responsible for helping families cope with life stressors?

Each chapter was peer reviewed, blind to authorship, by the series editorial board and other professionals knowledgeable about family stress and coping. A brief description of each chapter follows.

Overview of the Chapters

In Chapter 1, "Burnout as Systemic Traumatic Stress: A Model for Helping Traumatized Family Members," the editor reviews the family psychology and traumatology literatures and in particular those works which focus on secondary or systemic effects of trauma. Drawing from these sources of information, and building upon earlier theories, the editor suggests a model of systemic traumatic stress. At the heart of this model are the concepts of empathy and empathic contagion associated with systematic exposure to traumatic material. Together they lead to various forms of burnout that become more and more difficult to treat before interpersonal and legal divorce is inevitable.

In Chapter 2, "Understanding the Secondary Traumatic Stress of Children," Arlene Steinberg addresses the secondary traumatic impact on children witnessing directly or indirectly trauma to parents, siblings, or friends. Steinberg observes that this area has been neglected, as was the impact of traumatic experiences on children who were themselves victims. Witnessing may include observing or merely knowing that a loved one experienced a trauma. Children of victims, having experienced their parents' symptomatology without themselves undergoing the trauma, consistently display symptoms of burnout and STS: intrusion, hyperarousal, and enactments similar to their parents.

In Chapter 3, "Understanding the Secondary Traumatic Stress of Spouses," Kathleen Gilbert suggests that STS can be seen as "the stress of caring too much." She suggests that spouses may be at particular risk of the effects of STS because of the especially close, often emotionally intense nature of the spousal relationship. According to Gilbert, STS may be the result of direct (i.e., proximal) or indirect (i.e., distal) exposure to the primary victimization of one's spouse. Spouses also may experience a type of resonating STS reaction in which one partner's STS response acts as a trigger for the other's STS response. The development of STS responses in spouses results from their need to make sense of their partner's traumatic experience, and its aftermath is complicated by their efforts to maintain a stable and workable dyadic relationship. This may cause the secondarily affected spouse to become overresponsible and to overfunction for the primarily affected spouse. Efforts to protect may result in overprotection and isolation. Given the nature of the relationship, recovery requires that the partners learn new ways of thinking, new skills, new behaviors, and new interfactional patterns within the marital context. Therefore, the therapeutic plan for these couples should incorporate both individual and relationship issues.

In Chapter 4, "Understanding the Secondary Traumatic Stress of Parents," Michael F. Barnes focuses on the traumatization of parents following some type of physical traumatic event. It is estimated that 20,000 children die and another 100,000 are injured annually due to incidents associated with falls, automobile accidents, sports injuries, gunshot wounds, and related mishaps. Barnes proposes that while these injured children are traumatized, their family members experience both a secondary traumatization and a systemic traumatization that impact family functioning. The chapter reports on a comprehensive review of the literature associated with parental traumatization, adult traumatization, and related child-based medical literature. Finally, Barnes presents a set of axioms that were identified in the literature, which he proposes as the foundation for future research and treatment in this area.

In Chapter 5, "Treating STSD in Children," Mary Beth Williams focuses on promising treatment programs for the children of parents and others close to children who were *indirectly* traumatized, such as witnessing family violence, neighborhood violence, death, and other life experiences. Williams examines the impact of those stressors on children over the life span, from preschool to school age to preadolescent to adolescent. Further, she describes the general developmental level of each of these groups of children and then highlights the secondary symptoms that are age appropriate for each group. Next, she examines three specific areas of treatment: school-based interventions, individual treatment, and treatment for children who are secondarily traumatized within their own families of origin by exposure to parents who are trauma survivors and exhibit PTSD.

Chapter 6, "Treating Traumatized Partners: Producing Secondary Survivors of PTSD," Rory Remer and Robert A. Ferguson address the treatment of STSD in the partners of trauma victims. First, the phenomena of STSR and STSD are briefly defined and related to the concepts of primary and secondary victimization. Second, the authors present and discuss their model of secondary survivor healing, based on their previous work. It is based on working with partners of sexual assault victims and related to P. Remer's (1984) model of a primary survivor's healing processes. Third, Remer and Ferguson note the interface between the two models/processes, as well as its implications. Treatment interventions are presented and reviewed in light of both clinical experience and relevant research and are made along two dimensions: treatment goals (education, personal awareness/development, and skill acquisition) and a therapeutic milieu (individual, conjoint, or group therapy). Finally, the authors focus on several essential treatment issues: (1) alcohol/substance abuse, (2) preexisting pathology, (3) abusive partners, (4) individualizing approaches, (5) STSD primary victims, (6) helping vs. overinvolvement, (7) multiple therapeutic interventions, (8) impact on the therapist, and (9) balance between primary and secondary victim needs.

In Chapter 7, "Treating Burnout in Families Following Childhood Trauma," Michael F. Barnes focuses on two models of family therapy that can be effectively utilized to treat parents and other family members in a family in which a child has been traumatized. Barnes proposes that families experience alterations in both their organizational structure and in individual and family world view. He proposes that a Minuchin structural family therapy treatment approach be used initially. This approach, he argues, establishes the therapy environment as a safe place for the discussion of painful trauma memories. Once the therapeutic relationship has been developed, Figley's Family Empowerment Model is used to assist families to resolve conflicts associated with the traumatic event and to develop a healing theory to enable family members to recognize the strengths that allowed them to survive and move on with their lives.

In Chapter 8, "Treating Traumatized Families," Donald R. Catherall applies the model of recovery from individual traumatization to the burned-out environment of traumatized families. The focus is on specific aspects of the family environment which go awry as a consequence of traumatization. These elements become dysfunctional patterns in the family's intimate life, perpetuating a family environment in which the members are emotionally isolated and disconnected from one another. These effects are then passed along through the generations as a legacy of the family's traumatic past. The goal of the chapter is to provide clinicians with clearly defined areas of focus for family treatment sessions. Catherall breaks these sessions down into three categories. Within the category of disrupted caretaking, he identifies the parentification of children and the emotional inaccessibility of parents. Within the category of cognitive distortions, he focuses on family myths, a distorted world view, and the dysfunctional trauma issues, including reenactments, safety problems, the survivor missions taken on by many children, and the stressful presence of a family member with PTSD. Finally, Catherall emphasizes the importance of the therapist being personally authentic and conducting the seasons according to the standards of open communication.

CLOSING

This book is the first of several that will draw attention to the special vulnerabilities of families in which one or more members are exposed to chronic and acute stress. Subsequent books will deal with the psychology of interpersonal burnout resulting from everyday strains and stressors. This book focuses on the more extraordinary stressors, such as the death of a child, rape, life-threatening injury, and other stressor events. Using these events as markers, the chapters focus on how families tend to organize and reorganize around the catastrophe to both cope as individuals and enable the family to manage all of the various daily tasks.

This book contributes not only to the field of traumatology but also to the fields of family psychology and family therapy. Collectively, the chapters in this book suggest that psychologists and family therapists need to more fully explore the systemic fallout of traumatic events. Unless action is taken, there is a deterioration in the bonds that hold individuals together in intimate relationships. Not unlike measures taken by employers to keep their workers happy, motivated, and focused, we must take steps to keep our marriages and families happy, motivated, and focused. Family professionals are in the best position to help families avoid burnout and the stressful experiences and actions that lead to family burnout.

ACKNOWLEDGMENTS

This book emerged, in part, from the support of my family: Marilyn, Jessica, and Laura who are a source of inspiration.

Florida State University provided the critical home for my efforts to bring this project to fruition. Of special note is the support I received from the Interdivisional PhD Program; Dianne Montgomery, Dean of the School of Social Work; and Penny Ralston, Dean of the Interdivisional PhD Program and College of Human Sciences. The Editorial Board and outside reviewers deserve appreciation and are further recognized throughout the book.

REFERENCES

American Psychiatric Association (1994). *Diagnostic and statistical manual of mental disorders* (4th ed.). Washington, DC: American Psychiatric Association.

Burr, W. R. (1973). *Theory construction and the sociology of the family*. New York: John Wiley & Sons.

Figley, C. (1982). Traumatization and comfort: Close relationships may be hazardous to your health. Keynote presentation at Families and Close Relationships: Individuals in Social Interaction, conference held at Texas Tech University, Lubbock, February.

Figley, C. (1983). Catastrophes: An overview of family reactions. In, C.R. Figley and H.I. McCabbin (Eds.), *Stress and the Family*, Vol. 2: *Coping with Catastrophes*. New York: Brunner/Mazel, 3–20.

Figley, C.R. (1989). *Helping traumatized families*. San Francisco: Jossey-Bass.

Figley, C.R. (Ed.) (1995). *Compassion fatigue: Coping with secondary traumatic stress disorder in those who treat the traumatized*. New York: Brunner/Mazel.

Freudenberger, H.J. (1974). Staff burnout. *Journal of Social Issues, 30*(1), 159–165.

Hill, R., & Hansen, D. (1965). The family in disaster. In G. Baker and D.S. Chapman (Eds.), *Man and society in disaster* (pp. 37–51). New York: Basic Books.

Lavee, Y. (1985). *Family types and family adaptation to stress: Integrating the Circumplex model of family systems and the family adjustment and adaptation response model*. Unpublished doctoral dissertation. St. Paul: University of Minnesota.

Maslach, C. (1976). Burn-out. *Human Behavior, 5*(9), 16–22.

McCubbin, H.I., & McCubbin, M. (1989). Theoretical orientation to family stress and coping. In C.R. Figley (Ed.), *Treating stress in families* (pp. 3–43). New York: Brunner/Mazel.

McCubbin, H.I., Thompson, A., Pirner, P., & McCubbin, M.A. (1988). *Family types and family strengths: A life-span and ecological perspective*. Minneapolis: Burgess.

Olson, D.H., McCubbin, H.I., Barnes, H., Larsen, A., Muxen, M., & Wilson, M. (1983). *Families: What makes them work*. Newbury Park, CA: Sage.

Pines, A.M. (1993). Burnout. In L. Goldberger and S. Breznitz (Eds.), *Handbook of stress: Theoretical and clinical aspects* (2nd ed.) (pp. 386–402). New York: The Free Press.

Pines, A.M., & Aronson, E. (1988). *Career burnout: Causes and cures*. New York: The Free Press.

Reuben, R. (1949). *Families under stress*. New York: Harper & Row.

Selye. H. (1956). *The stress of life*. New York: McGraw-Hill.

Selye, H. (1974). *Stress without distress*. Philadelphia: Lippincott.

Solomon, Z. (1989). A three year prospective study of PTSD in Israeli combat veterans. *Journal of Traumatic Stress, 2*(1), 59–73.

Solomon, Z., Mikulincer, M., Fried, B., & Wosner, Y. (1987). Family characteristics of PTSD: A follow-up of Israeli combat stress reactions casualties. *Family Process, 26*, 283–294.

Solomon, Z., Waysman, M., Avitzur, E., & Enoch, D. (1991). Psychiatric symptomatology among wives of soldiers following combat stress reactions: The role of the social network and marital relations. *Anxiety Research, 4*, 213–223.

Solomon, Z., Waysman, M., Belkin, R., Levy, G., Mikulincer, M., & Enoch, D. (1992). Marital relations and combat stress reactions; the wives' perspective. *Journal of Marriage and the Family, 54*, 316–326.

BURNOUT AS SYSTEMIC TRAUMATIC STRESS: A MODEL FOR HELPING TRAUMATIZED FAMILY MEMBERS

Charles R. Figley, Ph.D.

The field of traumatology has inadvertently ignored a large segment of traumatized people: the family and other supporters of "victims." In other words, we have ignored those suffering in their own right as a result of a loved one being traumatized (Figley, 1982, 1983). This suggests that there is a kind of transmission of trauma from the victim to the supporters; this phenomenon is described as "compassion stress," and the most negative consequences of this stress result in "compassion fatigue" (Figley, 1995).

This chapter reviews the relevant literature that emphasizes the emotional costs of caring for the traumatized and offers a theoretical model. The model both accounts for the current findings and provides a blueprint for designing methods of research to test the model and ways of both treating and preventing compassion fatigue.

REVIEW OF THE LITERATURE ON SYSTEMIC STRESS

Historical and Theoretical Foundations

Among the first efforts to recognize the role of the transmission of traumatic material from one family member to another was the classic

1-57444-047-0/98/$0.00+$.50

study of World War II veterans' families by Hill (1949). Hill originated the concept of family stress. He was the first to suggest that the system of the family is greatly affected by crisis events such as war and post-war reunion.

Traumatology, the study of traumatic stress, has literally been invented in the last decade. Even though the origin of the study of human reactions to traumatic events can be traced to the earliest medical writings in *Kunus Pyprus* published in 1900 B.C. in Egypt (Veith, 1968; Trimble, 1985; Figley, 1989a), the justification for a field of study and treatment emerged only recently (Figley, 1988).

Several factors suggest the need for systematic study and treatment of trauma and its sequelae. One factor is increased public and professional awareness of the frequency of traumatic events and their extraordinary impact on people.

The DSM-III included the diagnosis of post-traumatic stress disorder (PTSD) (APA, 1980). Common symptoms experienced by a wide variety of traumatized persons were then viewed as a legitimate disorder that could be diagnosed and treated. The number of professionals working with traumatized people (including lawyers, therapists, emergency professionals, and researchers) grew, as did the accumulation of empirical research that validated the disorder.

The last 20 years has yielded research on the many types of traumatic events and the immediate and long-term consequences not only for those directly affected by the events (cf., Figley, 1978) but also for those indirectly affected as a result of knowing, living with, loving, or working with these "victims" (e.g., Figley & Lewis, 1978; Figley, 1989a). The new field of traumatology has made significant breakthroughs recently in understanding this process at the first world conference on traumatology (Figley, 1992c; Hobfoll, 1992). However, many family therapists may not be aware that the same principles which would predict that a spouse or child of a traumatized person is at risk of being traumatized also apply to them.

Burnout vs. Secondary Traumatic Stress Disorder

The term "burnout" was coined by Freudenberger (1976) nearly 20 years ago. According to Pines and Aronson (1988, p. 9), burnout is "a state of physical, emotional and mental exhaustion caused by long term involvement in emotionally demanding situations."

In contrast to burnout, which emerges gradually and is a result of emotional exhaustion, secondary traumatic stress disorder (STSD) can emerge suddenly without much warning. In addition to a faster onset of symptoms, Figley (1995) has noted that with STSD, in contrast to burnout, there is a sense of helplessness and confusion and a sense of isolation from supporters; the symptoms are often disconnected from real causes, and yet there is a faster rate of recovery from symptoms.

Studies of Vietnam Veterans' Families with STSD

Although the causal relationship between family dysfunction and war experiences is not clear, research focusing on the families of Vietnam veterans shows a pattern. Among other things, the war reverberates within these family systems long after the war is over, and those families with veterans suffering from PTSD are fundamentally different than those without a veteran family member who is suffering from PTSD (Figley & Kleber, 1995; Figley, 1995).

Carroll, Foy, and Donahoe (1985) found that the families of Vietnam combat veterans with PTSD were fundamentally different from other families. War veterans' families with PTSD had more marital problems, in terms of self-disclosure and expressiveness, hostility and aggression toward partners, and global marital maladjustment.

Similarly, Rueger (1983) found that the wives of Vietnam combat veterans were less communicative, more angry, and more fearful of their partners than comparison groups of wives of husbands who did not see combat. These findings are consistent with the approach advocated by Levy and Neuman (1987), who found that treatment of combat reactions was made more effective by involving families. These findings were generally confirmed by Verbosky and Ryan (1988) and Maloney (1988).

The most important study of families of war veterans was actually mandated by the U.S. Congress in 1983, through Section 102 of Public Law 980-160. It called for the study of Vietnam veterans to include "an evaluation of the long-term effects of postwar psychological problems among Vietnam veterans on the families of such veterans (and on persons in other primary social relationships with such veterans)" (Kulka, Schlenger, Fairbank, Hough, Jordan, Marmar & Weiss, 1990).

To follow this directive, the research team selected to conduct the study from the Research Triangle Institute, North Carolina organized the National Vietnam Veterans Readjustment Study. This study was viewed as the most comprehensive and definitive by both scientists and policymakers (Cranston, in Kulka et al., 1990). The team, following the most rigorous of epidemiological methodology, conducted 3,016 interviews of Vietnam war theater veterans matched by race, age, and gender with non-theater veterans and non-veterans. Among the findings:

- Approximately 30.6% of all male Vietnam theater veterans have or had PTSD at some time in their lives. This represents about 960,000 of the 3.14 million men who served in the war theater.
- Approximately 26.0% of all female Vietnam theater veterans have or had PTSD at some time in their lives. This represents about 1,900 of the 7,200 women who served in the war theater.
- Approximately 15.2% (479,000) of all male Vietnam (theater) veterans had PTSD at the time of the study. However, only 8.5% of all female Vietnam veterans had PTSD at the time of the study.
- This compared to only 2.5% of all male and 1.1% of all female Vietnam era veterans who have PTSD and with 1.2% of all male and 0.3% of all female non-veterans have PTSD.
- Ethnicity plays a major role in the current PTSD prevalence rates: 27.9% among Hispanics and 20.6% among African-Americans, compared with 13.7% among whites and others.

The research team also interviewed 474 of the spouses/partners of Vietnam veterans. They were asked to "describe their own problems, as well as the problems of the veterans' children." (Kulka et al., 1990, p. 236). The research team admitted in the report of its findings that it could not definitively address the cause–effect issue. That is, that PTSD caused family burnout or vice versa.

> However, the similarities between spouses of veterans with and without PTSD suggest that the source of marital and family discord may well be PTSD and its associated problems (p. 237).

The study found that spouses and partners of Vietnam veterans who were diagnosed with war-related PTSD, when contrasted with those without such a diagnosis, have the following family characteristics: (1) the veteran is married more often, (2) the veteran is married fewer years, (3) higher estimates of PTSD in the spouse/partner, (4) higher rate of readjustment problems, (5) lower rate of life functioning, (6) higher rate of marital problems, (7) higher and more dangerous rate of family violence, (8) higher rate of childhood behavioral problems, (9) lower rate of subjective well-being among the partner/spouse, (10) higher rate of demoralization, and (11) higher rate of vulnerability to a nervous breakdown (Kulka et al., 1990). These disturbing findings are not only consistent with other research that has focused on Vietnam veterans' families but also parallel the findings in Israeli war veterans' families.

Israeli War Veterans' Families

Solomon, Mikulincer, Freid, and Wosner (1987) looked at family characteristics and PTSD in a follow-up study of Israeli combat stress reaction casualties. The study investigated the role of family status and family relationships in the course of combat-related PTSD. The data sources were medical records, questionnaires, and scale data for a sample of 382 Israeli soldiers who suffered a combat stress reaction episode during the 1982 war with Lebanon. One year after the war, married soldiers had higher rates of PTSD than did unmarried soldiers.

It is revealing to note that Solomon et al. (1987) also found higher rates of PTSD to be associated with low expressiveness, low cohesiveness, and high conflict in the families. This lends support to the notion of the deleterious impact of war-related PTSD on families and challenges the simplistic notion that the availability of a family does not automatically ameliorate the symptoms of PTSD. Without information about family functioning prior to the war, however, it is not possible to conclude that PTSD caused the dysfunction found among these families.

Solomon (1989) has noted the effect of combat-related PTSD on the family. Acknowledging that the literature on the detrimental effects of combat-related PTSD indicates guilt feelings, emotional withdrawal, and elevated levels of aggression in the returning veteran, Solomon predicted and found in her series of studies that veterans with PTSD have a greater negative effect on their families than veterans without PTSD.

Thus, a war veteran with PTSD found it difficult, perhaps even impossible, to fully resume or undertake his formal roles of father, husband, and breadwinner. Therefore, it was not surprising that Solomon (1989) found that the wives and children of these veterans show psychiatric symptoms themselves to a much greater degree than families of veterans who do not have PTSD. Subsequent research by Solomon and her colleagues (Solomon, Waysman, Avitzur & Enoch, 1991), for example, found that wives of soldiers with PTSD are much more likely to suffer from higher levels of psychopathology and social dysfunction than those married to soldiers without PTSD.

Also, Solomon, Waysman, Belkin, Levy, Mikulincer, and Enoch (1992) found that, over time, the marital relations of Israeli combat veterans who sustained PTSD were more conflictual, less intimate, less consensual, less cohesive, and were marked by less reported marital satisfaction than marriages of combat veterans without PTSD. Most recently, Solomon, Waysman, Levy, Fried, Mikulincer, Benbenishty, Florian, and Bleich (1992) found that wives of veterans with PTSD, in contrast to wives of veterans without PTSD, had impaired social relations in a broad range of contexts, from inner feelings of loneliness, through impaired marital and family relations and relations with the wider social network.

THE TRAUMA TRANSMISSION CONUNDRUM

Although we now know much more than ever about the least known traumatic stress—compassion stress and compassion fatigue—the most fundamental question remains a conundrum. How is it that the physiological and emotional arousal caused by traumatic stress for those in harm's way is *also* found among those who attend to loved ones in harm's way? Scholars and clinicians require a conceptualization that accurately describes the indices of traumatic stress for those experiencing indirect as well as those experiencing direct traumatic stress. Also, how did the traumatic material get there, and how can it be removed?

The Trauma Transmission Model, described elsewhere (Figley, 1992f, 1995) and depicted in Figures 1.1 and 1.2, suggests that members of systems, in an effort to generate an understanding about a member who is experiencing traumatic stress, are motivated to express empathy toward the troubled member. Supporters attempt to answer for themselves the five victim questions (Figley, 1982, 1983, 1989a): What happened? Why did it happen? Why did I act as I did then? Why have I acted as I have since? If it happens again, will I be able to cope?

These supporters try to answer these questions for the victim in order to change his or her behavior accordingly. Yet, in the process of generating new *information,* the system member *experiences* emotions that are strikingly similar to the victim's. This includes visual images (e.g., flashbacks), sleeping problems, depression, and other symptoms that are a direct result of visualizing the victim's traumatic experiences, exposure to the symptoms of the victim, or both. The terms most relevant to this process include cognizance, discernment, sensitivity, understanding, comfort, identify with, understand, approve, endorse, sanction, embrace, receive, welcome, abide, bear, endure, suffer, tolerate, accept, commiseration, pity, compassion, and sympathy. This model draws from all of the important research and theoretical literature that has contributed to understanding traumatic stress, interpersonal relationships (e.g., empathy studies), and worker burnout (especially Miller, Stiff & Ellis, 1988).

The model suggests that the "burnout" of secondary traumatic stress is due, in part, to one's empathic ability, actions toward the sufferer and the inability to find relief from our actions through disengagement, and a sense of satisfaction from helping to relieve suffering.

This component of the model (see Figure 1.1) illustrates how Compassion Stress is a function of six interacting variables. Compassion Stress is defined as *the stress connected with exposure to a sufferer.* Empathic Ability is defined as *the ability to notice the pain of others.* It is frequently the characteristic that leads people to choose the role of helper, especially as a social worker, counselor, or other type of professional helper. This ability is, in turn, linked to one's susceptibility to Emotional Contagion, defined as *experiencing the feelings of the sufferer as a function of exposure to the sufferer.* This is similar to the feeling of being "swept up" in the emotion of the victim(s).

This is the very essence of the feeling of compassion for another. Being a member of a family or other type of intimate or bonded

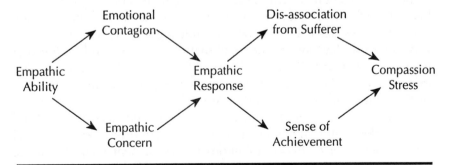

Figure 1.1   A Model of Compassion Stress

interpersonal relationship, we feel the pain (literally) of others. Much of this is associated, in turn, with identifying with a suffering loved one and feeling "for the grace of God go I."

Empathic Ability is also linked to Empathic Concern, defined as *the motivation to act to provide help.* Without the motivation to respond to the suffering family member, the helper does nothing—irrespective of the helper's ability to respond and the extent to which the helper is exposed to the suffering of the family member. Indeed, the lack of concern is a clear indicator of burnout of that family member.

Both Empathic Ability and Emotional Contagion account for the extent to which the person makes an effort to reduce the suffering of the sufferer. The effort is the Empathic Response. It is defined as *the right response, in tone, timing, temperament, and text, that helps the suffering family member, instance by instance.*

Efforts to help relieve the suffering take many forms and are assessed entirely in subjective terms by both the helper and the family member being helped. For a father, it is may be holding back giving a lecture or advice to a teenage daughter struggling through her first failed love relationship. For a mother, it may be the feeling of helplessness and lack of guidance when helping her son recover from the death of a good friend. For a sibling, it may be attempting to provide reassurance and hope to a younger sibling who must deal with being mistreated by friends.

What Makes a Difference in Increasing or Decreasing Compassion Stress?

Two major factors appear to make the difference. A Sense of Achievement is the extent to which the helping family member is satisfied with his or her efforts to relieve the suffering of the family member needing help. The other factor is Dis-Association from the suffering family member. It is the sense that one has done all that can be done and, in the best interest of everyone, living one's own life to the fullest without being forced to think about the suffering family member; it means "letting go" of the pain required to be compassionate.

Inevitably, the level of Compassion Stress experienced is associated with the degree to which the family member can dis-associate and feel satisfied with her or his contributions (Sense of Achievement). At the same time, in order to relieve the stress, some family members overestimate their Sense of Achievement and/or psychologically distance themselves more than necessary. These are also indicators of becoming burned out as a family member.

Conversely, those who experience very little Compassion Stress and yet are exposed to enormous Emotional Contagion and have considerable Empathic Ability and Empathic Concern find a sense of satisfaction in their Empathic Response because they believe they relieved suffering and, thus, have a Sense of Achievement or are able to avoid identifying with or becoming obsessed with the difficulties of the victim(s) and, thus, are effective at Distancing themselves psychologically from the sufferer. Sense of Achievement is satisfaction in reducing the suffering. Disengagement is separating self from sufferer personally and emotionally.

This second component of the trauma transmission model (see Figure 1.2) illustrates how Compassion Fatigue is a function of four interacting variables. Compassion Fatigue is defined as *a state of exhaustion and disfunction—biologically, psychologically, and socially—as a result of prolonged exposure to Compassion Stress and all that it evokes.* It is a form of burnout. In families, this can lead to family conflict, disruption, and even divorce.

Prolonged Exposure means an ongoing sense of responsibility for the care of the suffer and the suffering, over a protracted period of time. The sense of prolonged exposure is associated with a lack of relief from the burdens of responsibility, the inability to reduce the Compassion Stress. This variable has been recognized in long-term family care-givers, often adult daughters of the elderly who become "burned out" by the constant care requirements.

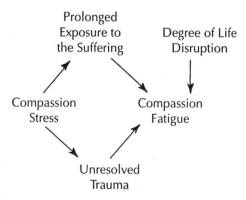

Figure 1.2   A Model of Compassion Fatigue

Traumatic Recollections are provoked by Compassion Stress and Prolonged Exposure. These recollections are of traumatic memories that stimulate the symptoms of PTSD and associated reactions, such as depression and generalized anxiety. In families, this can mean parents being reminded of childhood traumatic experiences triggered by their own children's current life crises (Figley, 1989a, 1989b).

Compassion Fatigue is inevitable if, added to these three factors, the family member under such enormous stressors experiences an inordinate amount of Life Disruption as a function of illness, change in life style, social status, or professional or personal responsibilities. This might be the "last straw" that leads to burnout, especially Compassion Fatigue.

On the other hand, such life crises may be an important antidote to the other stressors. For many family members who have a tendency to give to others in the family, a major life disruption may lead to a shift from providing care to receiving it. As a consequence, the family member not only avoids family burnout (Compassion Fatigue) but has endured another life challenge with the help of family members, including those who had received the member's help recently.

THE TREATMENT OF SYSTEMIC TRAUMATIC STRESS

Individuals such a war veterans have fairly extensive treatment program information available (cf., Kelly, 1985). Practice approaches and effectiveness in treating PTSD generally vary considerably. Some are more general and multiphasic treatment based on the individual progress of each client, like the programs to address and correct the compulsion to seek out life-threatening situations or "combat addiction." Some programs focus more specifically, such as those that adopt a cognitive/behavioral approach with direct exposure, implosion methods, various drug treatments, group psychotherapy, and hospital-based treatment. Other promising approaches provide even more specific procedures such as a focus on ethnicity or dual diagnosis of substance abuse and PTSD (Kuhn, Nohnber & Baraga, 1986; Schnitt & Nocks, 1984; Moyer, 1988).

However, few models are available for treating entire systems affected by trauma and the consequent Compassion Stress, Compassion Fatigue, and other forms of burnout from exposure to suffering members. The exceptions include the empowerment approach, proposed by Figley (1989a). Figley's model calls for families to come together to develop new skills and accepted practices that lead to more effective family supportiveness. In doing so, the family "practices" these new skills and approaches in discussing the sources of stress, stress reactions, methods of coping that were or were not useful and eventually developing a "healing theory" that helps the family members come to turns with and learn from the traumatic stressors that have affected them.

Models for families dealing with acute grief and sudden loss are noted by Figley, Bride, and Mazza (1997). Families grieve together over the death of a person significant to one or more family members, such as a parent or a grandparent. Families grieving the sudden and violent death are more challenged because prior to grief and loss accommodation there must be trauma accommodation: processing and working through the more frightening, gruesome, and disturbing aspects associated with the death first. A model recently developed by Therese A. Rando and Charles R. Figley (1996), depicted in Figure 1.3, illustrates this strategy well.

Another useful model which was originally developed for emergency workers and holds promise for families is called "debriefing." It is a form of crisis intervention that enables team members to discuss with candor what happened in response to a crisis and the emotional toll it has taken so far. Mitchell (1986, 1988) developed a model to help prevent emotional fallout from highly stressful or critical incidents. His critical incident stress debriefing has been adopted internationally to aid groups of emergency personnel work through and process troublesome duty-related events. These debriefings typically involve a group meeting of emergency workers immediately following the critical incident. The focus of the meeting is psychoeducational.

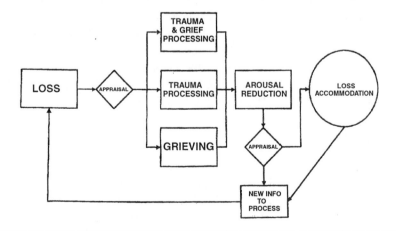

Figure 1.3   Traumatic Loss Accommodation

The goal is both to educate workers about secondary traumatic stress and to encourage group discussion regarding how the event affected each person personally.

Similarly, Everstine and Everstine (1983) apply a strategic therapeutic intervention approach to working with all types of groups and individuals, including couples and families. However, the emphasis is primarily on treating the traumatized rather than those who live with and care for them.

Fortunately, the chapters in this book fill a critical gap in the literature on secondary traumatic stress, compassion stress, and burnout among family members. As noted in the introductory chapter to this volume, Chapters 5 to 8 focus on treatment approaches for children, couples, parents, and families, respectively.

IMPLICATIONS FOR EDUCATING FAMILIES AND THOSE WHO CARE FOR THEM

We need to know much, much more about burnout in families and especially the systemic costs of trauma. We need to know who experiences compassion stress; for example, who gets it when and under what circumstances, and how it can be treated and prevented. However, we do know enough now to realize that family members are deeply affected by the suffering of other family members.

Recognizing this, family educators and policymakers have a special obligation to prepare traumatologists and related professionals who work with traumatized people to be especially sensitive to the family, friends, and other supporters of those in harm's way. We can start by incorporating stress, burnout, and STSD into our curriculum and especially our supervision in practica. We can utilize the relatively protected environment of our educational centers and the clients who seek help there as opportunities for discussing these issues in addition to the fundamental principles for preventing burnout.

REFERENCES

American Psychiatric Association (1980). *The Diagnostic and Statistical Manual of Mental Disorders, Rev III*. Washington, D.C.: Author.

Carroll, R., Foy, E., & Donahoe, S. (1985). Vietnam combat veterans with PTSD: Analysis of marital and cohabiting adjustment. *Journal of Abnormal Psychology*, 94: 329–337.

Everstine, D.S., & Everstine, L. (1983). *People in crisis: Strategic therapeutic interventions*. New York: Brunner/Mazel.

Figley, C.R. (1978). *Stress disorders among Vietnam veterans: Theory, research, and treatment.* New York: Brunner/Mazel.

Figley, C.R. (1982). Traumatization and comfort: Close relationships may be hazardous to your health. Keynote presentation at Families and Close Relationships: Individuals in Social Interaction, conference held at Texas Tech University, Lubbock, February.

Figley, C.R. (1983). Catastrophes: A overview of family reactions. In C.R. Figley and H.I. McCubbin (Eds.), *Stress and the family, Volume II: Coping with catastrophe* (pp. 3–20). New York: Brunner/Mazel.

Figley, C.R. (1988). Toward a field of traumatic stress. *Journal of Traumatic Stress, 1*(1), 3–16.

Figley, C.R. (1989a). *Helping traumatized families.* San Francisco: Jossey-Bass.

Figley, C.R. (Ed.) (1989b). *Treating stress in families.* New York: Brunner/Mazel.

Figley, C.R. (1992a). Posttraumatic stress disorder. Part I: Empirically based conceptualization and symptom profile. *Violence Update, 2*(7), 1; 8–11.

Figley, C.R. (1992b). Posttraumatic stress disorder. Part II: Relationship with various traumatic events. *Violence Update, 2*(9), 1; 8–11.

Figley, C.R. (1992c). Posttraumatic stress disorder. Part III: Relationship with various traumatic events, continued. *Violence Update, 2*(10), 1; 8–11.

Figley, C.R. (1992d). Posttraumatic stress disorder. Part IV: Generic treatment approaches. *Violence Update, 3*(3), 1;4;7–8.

Figley, C.R. (1992e). Posttraumatic stress disorder. Part V: Treatment approaches for specific traumatized groups. *Violence Update, 3*(4), 1;4;7–10.

Figley, C.R. (1992f). Secondary Traumatic Stress and Disorder: Theory, Research, and Treatment. Paper presented at the First World Meeting of the International Society for Traumatic Stress Studies, Amsterdam, June.

Figley, C.R. (Ed.) (1995). *Compassion Fatigue: Coping with Secondard Traumatic Stress Disorder in Those Who Treat the Traumatized.* New York: Brunner/Mazel.

Figley, C.R., Bride, B., & Mazza, N. (Eds.) (1997). *Death and Trauma: The Traumatology of Grieving.* London: Taylor & Francis.

Figley, C.R., & Kleber, R. (1995). Beyond the "victim": Secondary traumatic stress. In R. Kleber, C.R. Figley, and B.P.R. Gersons (Eds.), *Beyond trauma: Cultural and societal dynamics* (pp. 75–98). New York: Plenum.

Figley, C.R., & Lewis, D.W. (1978). Delayed stress response syndrome: Family therapy indications. *Journal of Marriage and Family Counseling, 4*(1), 53–60.

Freudenberger, H. (1980). *Burnout.* New York: Bantam.

Freudenberger, H.J. (1974). Staff burnout. *Journal of Social Issues, 30*(1), 159–165.

Hill, R. (1949). *Families under stress.* New York: Harper & Row.

Hobfoll, S. (1992). Conservation of resources and loss. Paper presented at the First World Conference of the International Society for Traumatic Stress Studies, Amsterdam, June.

Kelly, W.E. (Ed.) (1985). *Post-traumatic stress disorder and the war veteran patient.* New York: Brunner/Mazel.

Kulka, R.A., Schlenger, W.E., Fairbank, J.A., Hough, R.L., Jordan, B.K., Marmar, C.R., & Weiss, D.S. (1990). *Trauma and the Vietnam War Generation.* New York: Brunner/Mazel.

Levy, A. & Neuman, M. (1987). Involving families in the treatment of combat reactions. *Journal of Family Therapy, 9*(2), 177–188.

Maloney, L.J. (1988). Post traumatic stresses on women partners of Vietnam veterans. *Smith College Studies in Social Work, 58*(2), 122–143.

Miller, K.I., Stiff, J.B., & Ellis, B.H. (1988). Communication and empathy as precursors to burnout among human service workers. *Communication Monographs, 55,* 9.

Mitchell, J.T. (1986). Critical incident stress debriefing. *Response!* 24–25.

Mitchell, J. (1988). *Critical incident debriefing: A handbook.* Bowie, Maryland: Chevron Press.

Moyer, M.A. (1988). Achieving successful chemical dependency recovery in veteran survivors of traumatic s*tress. Alcoholism Treatment Quarterly, 4*(4), 19–34.

Pines, A.M., & Aronson, E. (1988). *Career burnout: Causes and cures.* New York: The Free Press.

Rando, T.A., & Figley, C.R. (1996). Trauma and Loss Workshop, Toronto, December 13.

Remer, R., & Ferguson, R.A. (1991). *Becoming a secondary survivor of sexual assault.* Unpublished manuscript.

Rueger, D.B. (1983). PTSD: Analysis of female partners' relationship perception. Paper presented at the annual meeting of the American Psychological Association, Anaheim, CA.

Schnitt, J.M., & Nocks, J.J. (1984). Alcoholism treatment of Vietnam veterans with PTSD. *Journal of Substance Abuse Treatment, 1*(3), 179–189.

Solomon, A., Benbenishty, R., & Mikulincer, M. (1991). The contribution of War-time, Pre-war, and Post-war factors to self-efficacy: A longitudinal study of combat stress reactions. *Journal of Traumatic Stress, 4*(3), 345–362.

Solomon, A., Mikulincer, M., Freid, B., & Wosner, Y. (1987). Family characteristics and PTSD: A follow-up of Israeli combat stress reaction casualties. *Family Process,* 383–394.

Solomon, Z. (1989). A three-year prospective study of PTSD in Israeli combat veterans. *Journal of Traumatic Stress, 2,* 59–73.

Solomon, Z., Waysman, J., Avitzur, E., & Enoch, D. (1991). Psychiatric symptomatology among wives of soldiers following combat stress reaction: The role of the social network and marital relations. *Anxiety Research, 4,* 213–223.

Solomon, Z., Waysman, M., Belkin, R., Levy, G., Mikulincer, M., & Enoch, D. (1992). Martial relations and combat stress reaction: The wives perspective, *Journal of Marriage and the Family, 54,* 316–326.

Solomon, Z., Waysman, M., Levy, G., Fried, B., Mikulincer, M., Benbenishty, R., Florian, V., & Bleich, A. (1992). From front line to home front: A study of secondary traumatization. *Family Process,* 31, 289–302.

Trimble, M.R. (1985). *Post-traumatic neurosis: From railway spine to the whiplash.* Chichester, UK: John Wiley.

Veith, I. (1968). *Hysteria: The history of a disease.* Chicago: University of Chicago Press.

Verbosky, S.J. & Ryan, D.A. (1988). Female partners of Vietnam veterans: Stress by proximity. *Issues in Mental Health Nursing, 9*(1), 95–104.

UNDERSTANDING THE SECONDARY TRAUMATIC STRESS OF CHILDREN

2

Arlene Steinberg, Psy.D.

INTRODUCTION

This chapter addresses the secondary traumatic impact of witnessing directly or indirectly trauma to parents, siblings, or friends. This area has been neglected, as had been the impact of traumatic experiences on children who were themselves victims. Witnessing may include observing or merely having the knowledge that a loved one experienced a trauma. Children of victims, having experienced their parents' symptomatology without themselves undergoing the trauma, have reportedly demonstrated the post-traumatic symptoms of intrusion, hyperarousal, and enactments similar to those of their parents. Writers have reported on the contagious effect of trauma (Terr, 1981b; Blom, 1986). Parental reactions may play a great role in the child's experience, at times determining the latter's reaction to the traumatic event, even for children directly traumatized. These observations highlight the interpersonal nature of trauma and may help explain the transmission of post-traumatic stress to offspring who were spared the actual traumatic experiences. Differences based on age, sex, and ethnicity, while pre-

1-57444-047-0/98/$0.00+$.50

liminary, are noted. The child's resilience and available supports can also modify the impact. The diagnostic category of secondary traumatic stress contextualizes the symptomatology of these children. Some implications of this diagnosis for assessment and treatment are discussed.

The literature of post-traumatic stress is remarkable for its paucity of references to the impact of trauma on children of victims. Even the effects of trauma on children who were direct victims have been neglected. Benedek (1985) notes the reactions in a professional meeting when the results of an important study on the child victims of the Chowchilla bus kidnapping were presented. She described the criticisms and concerns about overanalyzing and overdiagnosing. Perhaps it is a common resistance to not wish to see children tainted and terrorized by trauma. Indeed, if there is hesitance to acknowledge the traumatic impact on children who directly experience catastrophe and disaster in their own lives, then the denial of the less obvious impact of witnessing the trauma of a loved one is not surprising.

Children have been described as being profoundly affected and even experiencing post-traumatic symptomatology as a result of both directly witnessing the trauma of their loved ones (Nader, Pynoos, Fairbanks & Frederick, 1990; Pynoos & Eth, 1985) or by having knowledge that their family member (Rosenheck & Nathan, 1985) or friend experienced trauma (Blom, 1986; Parker, Watts & Allsopp, 1995). Living with parents who experience the flagrant symptomatology of post-traumatic stress disorder (PTSD), as a result of the traumatic experience of Vietnam or the Holocaust, has also resulted in the transmission of these symptoms to the next generation. The children too exhibit the intrusive symptoms and the hyperarousal of the disorder (Axelrod, Schnipper & Rau, 1980; Epstein, 1982). They may even share many of the same memories and reenact past parental traumatic experiences in their own lives without having the direct experiences.

This chapter describes the secondary traumatic impact of witnessing the trauma of parents, siblings, and friends either directly or indirectly. In addition, characteristics that account for the development or preventability, and that determine the presentation of post-traumatic stress among these children, are discussed. The issue of the possible mechanisms of transmission to the next generation is also addressed.

While children's victimization by war has been described (Freud & Burlingham, 1942; Freud & Dann, 1951; Solomon, 1942), the traumatic impact of disaster and criminal victimization on children only began to be addressed in the literature in the 1950s and beyond (Bloch, Silber

& Perry, 1956). As the advent of violence, war, and disaster is not new to the middle of the century, it appears that these children have been neglected.

DEVELOPMENT OF SECONDARY TRAUMATIC STRESS IN CHILDREN

There are two ways that children can develop secondary traumatic stress: either through witnessing their loved ones undergo traumatic experiences or merely by the knowledge that these significant others were traumatized, and perhaps living with the aftermath of the victim's nightmares, violence, anxiety, or other symptoms. The literature addresses these various situations; however, in many cases, it is difficult to tease them out. For instance, during wartime, children may both witness loss and devastation and also be aware of their parents' experiences in prison away from them. In situations of criminal victimization, the child may have both witnessed the violence to or violation of a parent and/or lived with the ensuing pain that the parent then feels. If the parent dies as a result, the child may become a more direct victim.

THE CHILD AS WITNESS

Freud (1918) was the first to address the profound influence on children's lives of witnessing; he focused on the primal scene, which he deemed traumatic. More recently, Pynoos and Eth (1985) described the symptomatology of children who witness the homicide, rape, or suicidal behavior of parents. As the rate of violent crimes has increased during the past 20 years, children are frequently witnesses to violent events in the lives of their loved ones. These children are vulnerable to the catastrophic events of other family members, given their feelings of deep caring for them (Figley, 1983). In addition, the experience of witnessing the "blood and gore" indelibly imprints on their minds an image that cannot be erased (Pynoos & Eth, 1985; Malmquist, 1986; Black, Harris-Hendricks & Kaplan, 1992). Figley (1983) stated that all family members should be considered victims regardless of whether they or another were victimized.

Pynoos and Eth (1985) distinguish between the experiences of witnessing and direct victimization. They describe the helplessness and passivity of the child witness who has to watch or listen to the sights and sounds of violence. While the injured child may become absorbed with internal sensations of pain and may not experience symptomatology or react to the personal meaning of the event until perhaps a later time, the child witness is immediately faced with an awareness of the overwhelming danger to the parent and may develop symptoms right away. The child witness is less likely to dissociate or experience feelings of numbness or disbelief. Children may suffer from profound feelings of guilt or self-blame for not having done more, and they fantasize having intervened to prevent the event. In cases of attempted suicide, children may feel more intensely the need to protect parents from future attempts. Due to their preoccupation with the danger to the parent and the need for intervention, they may not entertain a realistic appraisal of their own jeopardy, which may continue in other situations long after the violent episode. Dreman and Cohen (1990) describe several cases of children whose parents died in terrorist attacks; they felt guilt over not having helped the parents more. They also acted out self-destructively.

Anthony (1986) has stated that the psychological needs of both child victims and witnesses are frequently overlooked. Nader et al. (1990), Blom (1986), and Allodi (1980) have found children at all levels of trauma exposure to be profoundly affected and afraid of reoccurrence.

INTERPERSONAL TRAUMA

The concept of secondary traumatic stress highlights the interpersonal nature of trauma. Terr (1981a, 1981b) has written of the contagious impact of trauma on other family members and peers. She observed that the family members of children who were kidnapped on their school bus in Chowchilla exhibited reactions that were similar to, albeit less intense than, those of the actual victim. She indicates that family members were traumatized by the realization that their children were missing and also helpless. She attributes parental traumatization to the strong identification between parents and child, resulting in parents putting themselves in their child's place and experiencing the trauma as their offspring did. Family members not present, including other children in the family as well as close friends of the children, may suffer from long-term emotional consequences that are potentially seriously disabling in the family (Pynoos & Eth, 1985; Blom, 1986; McFarlane, 1987a, 1987b; Parker, Watts & Allsopp, 1995).

Terr (1981b) has also described the contagious effect of the traumatic experiences of one child on his or her non-related age-mates. She considers the child's post-traumatic play as the mechanism of transmission, whereby youngsters include their classmates or friends in play that painfully depicts the traumatic event, anxieties, and fears. Pynoos and Eth (1985) describe the case of one seven-year-old girl who witnessed her father strangle her mother and then carry the body to the bedroom; she forced all her friends to play the "mommy game." In this game, the child instructed her friends to "play dead and I pick you up." Terr (1981b) described the post-traumatic symptomatology exhibited by these other children. It seems that feelings of closeness and identification with the traumatized youngster as well as exposure to the horrific details in play make them vulnerable to the trauma.

Blom (1986) describes the ripple effect of traumatic situations to the community in the case of a collapsed skywalk in Lansing, Michigan. Children who merely knew of the event without direct exposure experienced fears and anxieties, albeit less than direct victims did. In a situation of a sniper attack on a school, children would check on siblings to assure themselves that they were safe (Nader et al., 1990). Indeed, the farther away the child was from the attack, the greater the worry expressed about siblings.

The importance of closeness with peers as a way to work through trauma has been noted by Freud and Dann (1951) in their description of orphaned young child survivors of the Holocaust, whose closeness with each other ameliorated the post-traumatic impact and sense of loss endured during World War II. The children formed intense bonds with one another. In opposite fashion, the enacted traumatic experiences of one child may serve to traumatize other children.

The vulnerability of children to their parents' reactions appears to be a consistent theme in the literature. Freud and Burlingham (1942) found that the extent of children's anxieties in reaction to the bombing in London during World War II was associated with their parents' reaction rather than with their exposure to the bombing itself. Ziv and Israeli (1973) similarly observed children's reactions to bombardment on kibbutzim in Israel to be determined more by their parents' attitudes than by the intensity of the danger experienced. These findings of greater reactivity to parents' emotional state than to the danger situations themselves seem to be consistently observed not only during wartime (Solomon, 1942) but in disaster situations (Bloch, Silber & Perry, 1956; Newman, 1976; Green, Korol, Grace, Vary, Leonard, Gleser & Smitson-Cohen, 1991;

McFarlane, 1987a, 1987b), during political persecution (Allodi, 1980), and in situations where children are faced with the threat of nuclear disaster (e.g., Three Mile Island [Handford, Mayer, Mattison, Humphrey, Bagneto, Bixler & Kales, 1986]). The reactions of parents or significant others can influence the extent to which the child will be traumatized.

McFarlane (1987a, 1987b) found that the mother's responses to an Australian bushfire disaster were better predictors of the presence of post-traumatic phenomena in children than the children's direct exposure to the disaster. Children were particularly affected by the intrusive memories of the mother as well as by her changed pattern of parenting. Children who played games about the fire seemed to have mothers who were not coping well with their experiences. This is consistent with the studies by Newman (1976) and Green et al. (1991) of the Buffalo Creek Disaster victims. Newman described the case of Marie, who did not directly see the ravages of the flood, but appeared to be traumatized by her relationship with her anxious, traumatized mother, as depicted in her drawings. She suggested that parental anxiety coupled with an awareness of their parents' inability to save others may leave the children feeling particularly vulnerable and unprotected. This also implies that parental calmness as described by Freud and Burlingham (1942) may signify safety and protection to their offspring. Green et al. (1991), in their follow-up study of these flood survivors, found that the youngest and oldest (adolescents) groups of youngsters tended to be more affected by parents' reactions than the middle group. Galante and Foa (1986) similarly found child survivors of an earthquake in Italy to react more strongly when family members were affected.

Newman (1976) discusses the possible impact of parental anxiety on the unborn children of Buffalo Creek flood survivors. This is a theme that will emerge in later discussion of the children of Vietnam veterans and Holocaust survivors.

While most of these studies have dealt with children who were themselves victimized by disaster or catastrophe, the observation that parental reactions played a great role in children's experiences highlights the extent to which traumatic experiences are interpersonal events. In addition, children's greater reactivity to their significant others than to the experienced traumatic events suggests that children who are not victims but are witnesses and even those born in the next generation may be affected to the extent that their parents are. The introduction of the concept of secondary traumatic stress highlights the interpersonal nature of trauma, such that children, so far as they care about parents, siblings, friends, and others, may come to be traumatized themselves.

While some writers (Blom, 1986; Nader, Pynoos, Fairbanks & Frederick, 1990) tried to differentiate the extent of traumatization based on proximity, the extent of traumatic exposure, or degree of personal life threat (Martini, Ryan, Nakayama & Ramenofsky, 1990; Green et al., 1991; Lonigan, Shannon, Taylor & Finch, 1994; Pynoos, Goenjian, Tashjian & Karakashian, 1993), others (Epstein, 1982; Axelrod, Schnipper & Rau, 1980; Rosenheck & Nathan, 1985; Eth & Pynoos, 1985) do not. Further research is needed to assess the extent to which proximity is a variable affecting extent of traumatization. Empathic involvement and identification with the victim can lead to post-traumatic symptoms that are as severe as the victim's own. Some of these issues are addressed in the next section.

SECONDARY TRAUMATIZATION: THE TRANSMISSION OF POST-TRAUMATIC STRESS TO THE NEXT GENERATION

The literature has begun to address the transgenerational effects of trauma with certain populations. In this section, transgenerational issues and mechanisms of transmission are examined. These issues can be seen as a type of chiasmal effect (Figley, 1985) whereby individuals in the next generation come to experience the post-traumatic symptoms of their parents, while never having experienced the trauma themselves. Post-traumatic symptoms have been observed among children of Holocaust survivors (Epstein, 1982; Axelrod, Schnipper & Rau, 1980), children of Vietnam veterans (Rosenheck & Nathan, 1985), children of Japanese-American internees in World War II (Nagata, 1990), and children of American and Canadian World War II veterans (Rosenheck, 1986).

Rosenheck and Nathan (1985) have termed this phenomenon secondary traumatization. They observed that among the offspring of male Vietnam veterans, the children relive their fathers' experience and may become obsessed with war-related concerns that trouble the veteran. These children may manifest symptoms similar to their fathers', including nightmares and fears of death and injury. In one case described, Alan seemed to be "living in one of his father's flashbacks rather than his own reality."

This phenomenon was initially described among children of Holocaust survivors, who were one of the first groups of survivors' offspring to be observed in both clinical and research settings. They, like the children of Vietnam veterans, had not actually experienced the traumatic events in their own lives; however, they manifested many of the same symptoms and worries as their parents, and even demonstrated behavioral reenactments that bore a striking resemblance to their parents' wartime experiences. They seem to have been profoundly affected by their parents' traumatic experiences.

Steinberg (1989) in previous writing has described the array of symptomatology discussed in the literature. Survivors' children have been noted to present in clinical settings with depression, anxiety, phobias, guilt, and separation problems (Barocas & Barocas, 1973; Freyberg, 1980); have manifested similar dream imagery, phobic phenomena, and environmental misperception (Epstein, 1982); and have even experienced anniversary reactions resembling parental experience (Axelrod, Schnipper & Rau, 1980). Kestenberg (1982) described a child-of-survivor complex. She considered survivors' children to be a heterogeneous group who present with a constellation of features. She distinguishes between a complex and a syndrome and stresses that it would not be accurate to label a "survivor's child syndrome." However, she feels that most, if not all, display these features.

Some of these studies have documented behavioral problems and symptoms in the childhood of Holocaust survivors' children (Sigal & Rakoff, 1971); however, most observations are of survivors' children in adulthood. For some, the experiences of young adulthood or adulthood threaten to stir up the trauma, and their identities as survivors' children may leave them vulnerable to later traumatic stress. Solomon, Kotler, and Mikulincer (1988) describe a subgroup of survivors' offspring who are faced with combat situations while soldiers in the Israeli Defense forces. They found them to be more vulnerable to PTSD than control subjects. Feelings of survivor guilt as well as conflicts over aggression were exacerbated for them. They particularly experienced conflicts between the desire to release aggression and the internalized prohibition against killing. The vivid images of parents' victimization experiences are triggered. They may also experience feelings of self-blame and failure more acutely than combat veterans, given that they are also viewed as the redeemers and protectors of their parents.

The literature on children of Vietnam veterans affords the opportunity to observe the impact of secondary traumatization in childhood, while descriptions of Holocaust survivors and World War II veterans' children provide a glimpse of the longer-term impact of secondary traumatization. Matsakis (1988) describes Vietnam veterans' children as young as three or four years old hiding under beds upon hearing helicopters or airplanes flying overhead. Matsakis (1988) and Rosenheck (1986) do not consider secondary traumatization as an inevitable outcome for all veterans' children. Rosenheck, in his study of World War II veterans and their offspring, finds that the children who seem to have the closest relationships with their fathers may develop similar symptomatology. These children were intimately exposed to their fathers' rage, depression, guilt, loss of impulse control, nightmares, and flashbacks. Other possible outcomes may include serving as rescuers, which results from a strong sense of responsibility for their fathers rather than from an identification with them. Many of these children had siblings who were of the more involved group. Younger siblings tend to be aware and concerned about their fathers, but asymptomatic. The final group was those who seemed remote and less involved, perhaps as a result of having fathers who kept their wartime experiences hidden. Sigal and Rakoff (1976) found in a Canadian sample of World War II veterans differences between children based on sex. He observed that firstborn female offspring of veterans who were interned in Japanese camps seemed to fare worse than their siblings.

While the children who suffered from secondary traumatization were not intimately exposed to the realities of war in their own lives, they are described as having intense symptoms, as do their parents. These observations, coupled with the influence of parental anxieties on child disaster victims, suggest that the effects of the interpersonal nature of trauma, in terms of the great impact of parental reactions and experiences on children, may have a more profound effect than the child's actual proximity to the traumatic event. The impact of parental trauma on the future generations of other populations has been studied as well. Nagata (1990) studied the transgenerational consequence of the Japanese-American internment and observed a greater sense of vulnerability among these children.

While the vulnerability of family members to secondary traumatic stress has been attributed to their feelings of empathy and caring (Figley, 1983), the actual mechanisms of transmission have been only minimally considered. Rosenheck and Nathan (1985), Matsakis (1988), and McFarlane (1987a, 1987b) have attributed the symptoms of children to their exposure to parental morbidity and symptomatology. Rosenheck and Nathan describe the vulnerability of children exposed to their Vietnam veteran fathers' reliving experiences, leading to an identification with them and to the elaboration in the children's fantasy of the kind of event that the fathers had lived through. The parents' fears, memories, and reliving experiences can at times be quite frightening to the child (e.g., when Vietnam veterans react with violence during their flashbacks). At times, these reactions may coincide with the child's own experiences. Haley (1984) cites the example of a father's intense negative response to his preschool child's aggressive play, which stirred up memories of Vietnam. Solomon (1988) indicates that the "natural exuberance and aggressiveness of a growing child (especially a son) may reawaken memories of wartime aggression, and may provoke excessive rage or guilt over sadistic impulses" (p. 326).

Another mechanism of transmission has to do with the closeness between parents and children, as the latter were more likely to be traumatized when they experienced their fathers as their emotional center. In turn, these children were overvalued and overprotected (McFarlane, 1987a, 1987b). For some veterans and Holocaust survivors, the children came to symbolize dead relatives or friends, including a dead buddy or Vietnamese girlfriend. Holocaust survivors' children were frequently named after a dead relative and complained that they were often confused with their namesakes. These children were frequently overidentified not only with their parents but with the deceased (Trossman, 1968; Phillips, 1978; Roden & Roden, 1982; Rustin, 1980; Klein, 1973). Difficulties with separation are described for Holocaust survivors' offspring (Freyberg, 1980; Trossman, 1968; Barocas & Barocas, 1973; Klein, 1973), as well as for veterans' children, which may contribute to the child's greater identification with his/her parents' traumatic experiences (Rosenheck & Nathan, 1985). In addition, the importance of parents verbalizing affects and traumatic experiences, in order to detoxify the memories of traumatic experiences (Grinker & Spiegel, 1945; Rosenheck & Thomson, 1986) and reduce the likelihood of post-traumatic symptomatology in the next generation, has been discussed (Rosenheck & Thomson, 1986) and empirically supported (Cahn, 1987).

GENDER, AGE, AND CULTURAL INFLUENCES

The influence of the gender and age of the child on his/her secondary traumatization experience has been only minimally considered. Sigal and Rakoff (1976) found female firstborn children to be particularly vulnerable to secondary traumatization due to their close relationship and identification with mothers who seemed to carry the burden in these families. At the same time, the aggressive play of sons of combat veterans may be more threatening to their fathers than similar play of daughters (Solomon, 1988), leading to greater difficulty for male children.

Although studies of children of Holocaust survivors distinguish between the effects on children based on the age at which parents were traumatized, they do not address the impact of the child's own age on his or her experience. Studies (Green et al., 1991; Pynoos & Eth, 1985; Shannon, Lonigan, Finch & Taylor, 1994) of children who were direct victims observed differences between younger and older, with the former group displaying more behavioral disturbance than the latter, who experienced more psychological distress (Green et al., 1991; Pynoos & Eth, 1985). Yet others have found no differences between children based on age or sex (Nader, Pynoos, Fairbanks & Frederick, 1990). Further research is needed in order to assess whether sex and age differences are demonstrated in situations of secondary traumatic stress. Indeed, Green et al. (1991) found that the youngest and adolescent children are more sensitive to parental reactions. This may suggest increased vulnerability to secondary traumatic stress in these age groups, as these children are more likely to identify with and be affected by their parents' traumatic experiences.

It appears that children of all ethnicities and cultural groups are vulnerable to secondary traumatic stress. Sigal and Rakoff (1976) have stated that traumatic stress is sufficient to erase cultural and ethnic differences. Literature has shown that the families of American, Japanese, Israeli, Jewish, and non-Jewish survivors have manifested secondary traumatic stress. The literature has also addressed specific cultural influences. Scaturo and Hardoby (1988) found that Vietnam veterans whose fathers were blue-collar workers (many of whom were World War II veterans) grew up in a culture where the idea of distinguishing oneself in combat was more highly thought of than a professional career. Frequently, the experiences of these veterans upon returning home did not meet their expectations. They were not provided with the cultural means to reintegrate into society, instead experiencing rejection upon return. In contrast, the return of American Indian combat veterans to structured purifying rituals helped them cope with their experiences of killing, leading to a lower incidence of post-traumatic stress in this group. In another instance, Israeli children of Holocaust survivors have benefited from the national, ritualized Holocaust remembrances and have been described as faring better than their American counterparts (Klein, 1973).

The appearance of secondary traumatic stress is also influenced by the child's resilience, as well as by the available supports and structure following the traumatic experience. Child trauma victims seem to benefit from the availability of family and the quick return to daily routines (Galante & Foa, 1986). Malmquist (1986) among others (Martini et al., 1990) felt that children who had been exposed to earlier object losses in gradual doses dealt better with the major trauma of witnessing parental murder due to their ability to soothe themselves. These children were able to maintain a sense of their self-worth and value. McFarlane (1987a, 1987b) also discussed the importance of parents' ability to contain their offspring's anxieties in preventing post-traumatic stress in children. This may be particularly relevant for the children of victims, as the stressor they confront is parental anxiety.

ASSESSMENT AND TREATMENT IMPLICATIONS

The fact that the psychological needs of child witnesses and victims have been neglected may reflect problems with assessment and diagnosis. Holocaust survivors' children have been misdiagnosed as psychotic (Kestenberg, 1982), only to have their symptoms remit when striking resemblance of these to their parents' Holocaust experiences were considered. Other children have been underdiagnosed, given a need to deny their difficulties. Only with the classification of PTSD were the victims' symptoms and pain more consistently viewed within the context of their traumatization. Family members, particularly children, are only beginning to receive organized attention, so that they too can be helped. The diagnostic category of secondary traumatic stress disorder contextualizes their difficulty, thereby providing an organized way to view their symptoms.

Assessing secondary traumatic stress requires an in-depth evaluation of the child within the context of the family, including the details of the traumatic event that may be reenacted by the child. The use of projective techniques, including play and drawings, to elicit details and feelings about the traumatic episode has been discussed with regard to child victims. These methods may also be useful in work with child witnesses and children of victims as well. The importance of assessing children directly is underscored by observations that children tend to report their reactions more accurately than their parents. Injured parents may particularly need to deny or minimize the impact of their experiences on children due to feelings of guilt at having harmed them. Pynoos and Eth (1986) have provided an interview format to assess child victims individually; this may be adaptable for child witnesses and the second generation as well.

Both child witnesses and children of traumatized parents demonstrate not only similar symptoms but also fantasies of wishing to intervene in order to rescue their loved one. Treatment involving play-acting these rescue fantasies may reduce their feelings of helplessness (Pynoos & Eth, 1985). For children who have witnessed the traumatic event, early intervention may prevent later symptomatology (Dreman & Cohen, 1990). However, for children of veterans or survivors, early intervention may not apply, as the event did not occur in their lifetime.

Many writers stress the importance of the expression of emotion or abreaction in the treatment of trauma survivors (Grinker & Spiegel, 1945; Scaturo & Hardoby, 1988; Solomon, Mikulincer, Freid & Wosner, 1987). Rosenheck and Thomson (1986) also discuss this in the context of treating the victim and his family. Their treatment model includes an initial disjoint phase of treatment involving separate sessions with the veteran and each family member. This enables the veteran to more openly express his feelings and memories without feeling shame and fearing his family's reactions to his brutal actions. It also enables wives and children to express their own bitterness without hurting their husband/father. Family members are educated in individual sessions about the realities of war in general and Vietnam in particular. The child's learning basic facts about the war facilitates his/her differentiation from the father, as the details of the father's experiences contrast with the reality of the child's own life. Wives and children can also come to understand the context behind the violent acting out or the frightening nightmares and are therefore less afraid of these behaviors and symptoms. Rosenheck and Thomson (1986) state that "the disjoint phase provides psychological space within which they can gain distance from the intensity of family interaction and can begin to develop a cognitive mastery over issues central to their father's distress as well as their own" (p. 567), thus detoxifying war memories. Family members then have a greater understanding of the impact of war on all family members.

Many writers (Fogelman, 1989; Rosenheck & Thomson, 1986; Brown, 1984) have also recommended support groups, which universalize the experience, resulting in a greater feeling of being understood. This may be helpful for children, whose needs have in the past been minimized, if not denied. A support group could provide acknowledgment of their difficulties as well as a place to work through their complicated feelings and fantasies. While this method may appear to be more useful with older children and adolescents, the utility of an adapted version of this approach for young children may need to be addressed.

FUTURE DIRECTIONS

Studies have stressed the greater impact of parental reactions on the child's experience of traumatic stress over the child's actual exposure to the traumatic event. Indeed, one can even assume that it is this impact that leads to transgenerational effects. One wonders to what extent this is true for all groups of trauma victims and how long-lasting these effects are. Some literature suggests that children removed from the disaster situation are not as likely to have long-lasting symptoms as those who were more directly exposed (Nader et al., 1990). However, the literature on Holocaust survivors' and Vietnam veterans' children discusses the long-lasting effects of parental experience and symptoms on a group that appears to be quite removed from trauma. Further research is needed to clarify these discrepancies.

As not all children experience secondary traumatization, systematic investigation of the factors influencing which children are more affected is needed. Observations of the child's closeness with the traumatized parent as well as of parental difficulties with certain children (Haley, 1984; Solomon, 1988) have been noted; however, writers seem to disagree on which children are more likely to suffer (e.g., firstborn daughters of veterans [Sigal & Rakoff, 1976] or their sons [Haley, 1984; Solomon, 1988]). Future investigation may clarify the existence of differences based on the child's gender, particularly as some studies of child victims have found no sex differences (Nader et al., 1990). Perhaps the traumatization of these children is great enough to erase differences; however, for the second generation, who are more removed from the traumatization, these differences resurface. This would suggest that proximity and degree of exposure to the trauma are significant variables. Further research must clarify these issues as well as the influence of culture, ethnicity, and race. While many Vietnam veterans were African or Hispanic Americans, little mention has been made of the impact on minority group veterans and their children of their having fought a war for a country that rejected them upon their return.

REFERENCES

Allodi, F. (1980). The psychiatric effects in children and families of victims of political persecution and torture. *Danish Medical Bulletin, 27*(5), 229–232.

Anthony, E.J. (1986). The response to overwhelming stress: Some introductory comments. *Journal of the American Academy of Child Psychiatry, 25*(33), 299–305.

Axelrod, S., Schnipper, O.I., & Rau, J.H. (1980). Hospitalized offspring of Holocaust survivors. *Bulletin of the Meninger Clinic, 44*, 1–14.

Barocas, H., & Barocas, C. (1973). Manifestations of concentration camp effects on the second generation. *American Journal of Psychiatry, 130*(7), 820–821.

Benedek, E. (1985). Children and psychic trauma: A brief review of contemporary thinking. In S. Eth and R.S. Pynoos (Eds.), *Post-traumatic stress disorder in children* (pp. 3–16). Washington, DC: American Psychiatric Press.

Black, D., Harris-Hendricks, J., & Kaplan, T. (1992). Father kills mother: Post-traumatic stress disorder in the children. *Psychotherapy & Psychosomatics, 57*(4), 152–157.

Bloch, D.A., Silber, E., & Perry, S.E. (1956). Some factors in the emotional reactions of children to disaster. *American Journal of Psychiatry, 113*, 416–422.

Blom, G.E. (1986). A school disaster—instruction and research aspects. *Journal of the American Academy of Child Psychiatry, 25*(3) 336–345.

Brown, P.C. (1984). Legacies of war: Treatment considerations with Vietnam veterans and their families. *Social Work*, July–August, 372–379.

Cahn, A. (1987). *The capacity to acknowledge experience in holocaust survivors and their children*. Unpublished doctoral dissertation. Garden City, NY: Adelphi University.

Dreman, S., & Cohen, E. (1990). Children and victims of terrorism revisited. *American Journal of Orthopsychiatry, 60*(2) 204–209.

Epstein, A.W. (1982). Mental phenomena across generations: The Holocaust. *Journal of the American Academy of Psychoanalysis, 10*(4), 565–570.

Eth, S., & Pynoos, R. (1985). Developmental perspective on psychic trauma in childhood. In C.R. Figley (Ed.), *Trauma and its wake, Volume I* (pp. 36–52). New York: Brunner/Mazel.

Figley, C.R. (1983). Catastrophes: An overview of family reactions. In C.R. Figley and H.I. McCubbin (Eds.), *Stress and the family, Volume II: Coping with catastrophe* (pp. 3–20). New York: Brunner/Mazel.

Figley, C.R. (1985). From victim to survivor: Social responsibility in the wake of catastrophe. In C.R. Figley (Ed.), *Trauma and its wake, Volume I* (pp. 398–415). New York: Brunner/Mazel.

Fogelman, E. (1989). Group treatment of a therapeutic modality for generations of the Holocaust. In P. Marcus and A. Rosenberg (Eds.), *Healing their wounds* (pp. 119–133). New York: Praeger.

Freud, A., & Burlingham, D. (1942) *War and children*. Report 12 in the writings of Anna Freud, Volume 3. New York: International Universities Press, 1973.

Freud, A., & Dann S. (1951). An experiment in group upbringing. *Psychoanalytic Study of the Child, 6,* 127–169.

Freud, S. (1918). From the history of an infantile neurosis. In J. Strachey (Ed.), *The standard edition of the complete psychological works of Sigmund Freud, Volume 17.* London: Hogarth Press.

Freyberg, J. (1980). Difficulties in separation-individuation of experience by offspring and Nazi Holocaust survivors. *American Journal of Orthopsychiatry, 50*(1) 87–95.

Galante, R., & Foa, D. (1986). An epidemiological study of psychic trauma and treatment effectiveness for children of a natural disaster. *Journal of the American Academy of Child Psychiatry, 25*(3), 357–363.

Green, B., Korol, M., Grace, M., Vary, M., Leonard, A., Gleser, G., & Smitson-Cohen, S. (1991). Children and disaster: Age, gender and parental effects on PTSD symptoms. *Journal of the American Academy of Child and Adolescent Psychiatry, 30*(6), 945–951.

Grinker, R.R., & Spiegel, J.P. (1945). *Men under stress.* Philadelphia: Blackiston.

Haley, S. (1984). The Vietnam veteran and his preschool child: Child rearing as a delayed stress in combat veterans. *Journal of Contemporary Psychotherapy, 14,* 114–121.

Handford, M., Mayer, S., Mattison, R., Humphrey, F., Bagneto, S., Bixler, E., & Kales, J. (1986). Child and parent reaction to the Three Mile Island nuclear accident. *Journal of the American Academy of Child Psychiatry, 25*(3), 346–356.

Kestenberg, J. (1982). Psychoanalysis of children of survivors from the Holocaust. In M. Bergman and M. Jucovy (Eds.), *Generations of the Holocaust* (pp. 137–188). New York: Basic Books.

Klein, H. (1973). Children of the Holocaust: Mourning and bereavement. In E.J. Anthony and C. Koupernick (Eds.), *The Child in this family* (pp. 393–409). New York: John Wiley.

Lonigan, C., Shannon, M., Taylor, C., & Finch, A. (1994). Children exposed to disaster. II: Risk factors for the development of post-trauma symptomatology. *Journal of the American Academy of Child and Adolescent Psychiatry, 33*(1), 94–105.

Malmquist, C.P. (1986). Children who witness parental murder: Post-traumatic aspects. *Journal of the American Academy of Child Psychiatry, 25*(3) 320–325.

Martini, D., Ryan, C., Nakayama, D., & Ramenofsky, M. (1990). Psychiatric sequelae after traumatic injury: The Pittsburgh Regatta accident. *Journal of the American Academy of Child and Adolescent Psychiatry, 29*(1) 70–75.

Matsakis, A. (1988). *Vietnam wives.* Kensington, MD: Woodbine House.

McFarlane, A. (1987a). Post-traumatic phenomena in a longitudinal study of children following a natural disaster. *Journal of the American Academy of Child and Adolescent Psychiatry, 26,* 764–769.

McFarlane, A. (1987b). Family functioning and overprotection following a natural disaster: The longitudinal effects of post-traumatic morbidity. *Australian and New Zealand Journal of Psychiatry, 21,* 210–218.

Nader, K., Pynoos, R., Fairbanks, L., & Frederick, C. (1990). Children's PTSD reaction one year after sniper attack on their school. *American Journal of Psychiatry, 147*(11), 1526–1530.

Nagata, D. (1990). The Japanese American internment: Exploring the transgenerational consequences of traumatic stress. *Journal of the Traumatic Stress, 3*(1), 47–69.

Newman, C.J. (1976). Children of disaster: Clinical observations at Buffalo Creek. *American Journal of Psychiatry, 133*(3), 306–312.

Parker, J., Watts, H., & Allsopp, M.R. (1995). Post-traumatic stress symptoms in children and parents following a school-based fatality. *Child: Care, Health & Development, 21*(3), 183–189.

Phillips, R. (1978). Impact of Nazi Holocaust on children of survivors. *American Journal of Psychotherapy, 32,* 370–377.

Pynoos, R., & Eth, S. (1985). Children traumatized by witnessing acts of personal violence: Homicide, rape or suicidal behavior. In S. Eth and R. Pynoos (Eds.), *Post-traumatic stress disorder in children* (pp. 19–43). Washington, DC: American Psychiatric Press.

Pynoos, R., & Eth, S. (1986). Witness to violence: The child interview. *Journal of the American Academy of Child Psychiatry, 25*(3), 306–319.

Pynoos, R., Goenjian, A., Tashjian, M., & Karakashian, M. (1993). Post-traumatic stress reactions in children after the 1988 Armenian earthquake. *British Journal of Psychiatry, 163,* 239–247.

Roden, R., & Roden, R. (1982). Children of Holocaust survivors, *Adolescent Psychiatry, 10,* 66–72.

Rosenheck, R. (1986). Impact of post-traumatic stress disorder of WW II on the next generation. *Journal of Nervous and Mental Disease, 174*(6), 319–327.

Rosenheck, R., & Nathan, P. (1985). Secondary traumatization in children of Vietnam veterans. *Hospital and Community Psychiatry, 36*(5), 538–539.

Rosenheck, R., & Thomson, J. (1986). "Detoxification" of Vietnam war trauma: A combined family-individual approach. *Family Process, 25,* 559–570.

Rustin, S. (1980). The legacy is loss. *Journal of Contemporary Psychotherapy, 2*(1), 32–43.

Scaturo, D., & Hardoby, W. (1988). Psychotherapy with traumatized Vietnam combatants: An overview of individual, group and family treatment modalities. *Military Medicine, 153*(4), 262–269.

Shannon, M., Lonigan, C., Finch, A., & Taylor, C. (1994) . Children exposed to disaster. I: Epidemiology of post-traumatic symptoms and symptom profiles. *Journal of the American Academy of Child and Adolescent Psychiatry, 33*(1), 80–93.

Sigal, J., & Rakoff, V. (1971). Concentration camp survival: A pilot study of efforts on the second generation. *Canadian Psychiatric Association Journal, 16,* 393–397.

Sigal, J., & Rakoff, V. (1976). Effects of paternal exposure to prolonged stress on the mental health of the spouse and children. *Canadian Psychiatric Association Journal, 21,* 169–172.

Solomon, J. (1942). Reactions of children to blackouts. *American Journal of Neuropsychiatry, 12,* 361–362.

Solomon, Z. (1988). The effect of combat-related post-traumatic stress disorder on the family. *Psychiatry, 51,* 323–329.

Solomon, Z., Mikulincer, R., Freid, B., & Wosner, Y. (1987). Family characteristics and post-traumatic stress disorder: A follow-up of Israeli combat stress reaction casualties. *Family Process, 26,* 383–394.

Solomon, Z., Kotler, M., & Mikulincer, M. (1988). Combat-related post-traumatic stress disorder among second generation Holocaust survivors: Preliminary findings. *American Journal of Psychiatry, 145*(7), 865–868.

Steinberg, A. (1989). Holocaust survivors and their children: A review of the clinical literature. In P. Marcus and A. Rosenberg (Eds.), *Healing their wounds* (pp. 23–48). New York: Praeger.

Terr, L. (1981a). Psychic trauma in children: Observations following the Chowchilla school-bus kidnapping. *American Journal of Psychiatry, 138*(1), 14–19.

Terr, L. (1981b). Forbidden games—Post-traumatic child's play. *Journal of the American Academy of Child Psychiatry, 20,* 741–760.

Trossman, B. (1968). Adolescent children of concentration camp survivors. *Canadian Psychiatric Association Journal, 12,* 121–123.

Ziv, A., & Israeli, R. (1973). Effects of bombardment on the manifest anxiety level of children living in kibbutzim. *Journal of Consulting and Clinical Psychology, 40,* 187–201.

UNDERSTANDING THE SECONDARY TRAUMATIC STRESS OF SPOUSES

Kathleen Gilbert, Ph.D.

INTRODUCTION

Secondary traumatic stress (STS), in many ways, can be seen as the stress of caring too much. Spouses may be at particular risk for the effects of STS because of the especially close, often emotionally intense, nature of the spousal relationship. It may be the result of direct (i.e., proximal) or indirect (i.e., distal) exposure to the primary victimization of one's spouse. Spouses also may experience a type of resonating STS reaction in which one partner's STS response acts as a trigger for the other's STS response. The development of STS responses in spouses results from their need to make sense of their partner's traumatic experience and its aftermath. It is complicated by their efforts to maintain a stable and workable dyadic relationship. This may cause the secondarily affected spouse to become overresponsible and to overfunction for the primarily affected spouse. Efforts to protect may result in overprotection and isolation. Given the nature of the relationship, recovery requires that they learn new ways of thinking, new skills, new behaviors, and new interactional patterns. Therefore, the therapeutic plan for these couples should incorporate both individual and couple therapy.

1-57444-047-0/98/$0.00+$.50
© 1998 by CRC Press LLC

The couple serves as the basic building block of the family, the basic unit of reproduction, intimacy, and love (Blumstein & Schwartz, 1983). Spouses* are affected by a traumatic event, whether it impacts directly on both partners (e.g., a fire that destroys their home) or on only one partner (e.g., the wartime experience of the husband or the abduction and rape of the wife). The interactive nature of the spousal relationship, cultural norms, role expectations, and feelings of obligation all contribute to the susceptibility of spouses to experience each other's stress. In this chapter, the lives of individuals as they evidence symptoms of traumatic stress exposure that are the result of their spouse's traumatic stress experience are considered.

As defined in this volume, secondary traumatic stress disorder (STSD) is

> a syndrome of symptoms nearly identical to PTSD [post-traumatic stress disorder], except that exposure to knowledge about a traumatizing event experienced by a significant other is associated with the set of STSD symptoms, and PTSD symptoms are directly connected to the sufferer, the person experiencing primary traumatic stress (Figley, 1995, p. 8).

This is an anxiety disorder, traceable to another person's exposure to a traumatic event or series of events, images, and memories related to the trauma. Secondary traumatic stress response (STSR) is a less severe form of STSD. In contrast to the direct (primary) experience of a traumatic stressor (post-traumatic stress [PTS]), STS is the result of the supporter's efforts to empathize (i.e., to understand and "emotionally connect") with the primary victim. It may also result from inadvertent exposure to the PTS of the primary victim. In both cases, the STS-affected person needs to understand and predict the PTS victim's sometimes erratic behavior and emotional state.

Secondary traumatic stress is the stress of caring too much, and the continuing, emotion-laden relationship between husband and wife may cause spouses to develop a unique interactional pattern following the victimization (Ford et al., 1993). It has been described among professional care providers (Figley, 1995), and the recommendation has been

---

* Unless otherwise noted, the terms "spouse" and "partner" will be used generically to indicate both marital and non-marital partners. As was found in the literature reviewed, when researchers examined the impact of the partner's PTSD on both marital and non-marital partners, they found no difference in experience based on marital status (cf., Williams, 1980).

made that they limit the depth of their relationship with the victimized person (Corcoran, 1989). While it may be possible, and even desirable, for professionals to do this, such a restriction of involvement would be contrary to the nature of the spousal relationship.

STSD and STSR result from what Figley (1989) has referred to as "vicarious" or indirect secondary effects and the "chiasmal effect," a more direct exposure. Here, these two forms of STS will be referred to as distal (i.e., vicarious) and proximal (i.e., chiasmal effect) STS.

DISTAL AND PROXIMAL SECONDARY TRAUMATIC STRESS

Distal STS is a vicarious victimization that results from "events in the imagination" (Terr, 1989). It consists of the secondary effects of caring emotionally about one's spouse who is in a potentially life-threatening situation, physically distant, and out of regular contact with the partner. With distal STS, there is no way to confirm the health and well-being of the spouse; indeed, it may not even be possible to determine if the spouse is alive. The distal STS-affected spouse may feel a strong need to prepare for the return of the missing spouse, but has limited information regarding the nature and timing of that return. Spouses coping with distal STS would experience the stress of uncertainty: about their spouses' fate, about reorganizing their lives and those of their children, and about their relationships with others whose support may not have been what they had expected (Boss, 1987, 1991). Examples of spouses at risk for this type of STS would include the husband of a woman who has been kidnapped and the wife of a serviceman still listed as missing in action.

Proximal STS would be exemplified in the wife of a returned war veteran or the husband of a woman who has been raped and is attempting to cope with the long-term effects of her traumatization. In each of these cases, the supporting spouse experiences the stressors related to daily contact with his or her affected partner after the traumatic event. Resources are drained as the proximal STS-affected spouse is exposed to the other's depression, rage, isolation, sleeping problems, emotional numbing, flashbacks, etc. If other demands (e.g., children's need to understand and/or be protected) are placed on the spouse who is dealing with her or his own STS, and if limited outside resources are available, the supporting spouse may experience burnout. It should not be surprising that 38% of Vietnam veterans' marriages ended within six months of their return from Vietnam (President's Commission on Mental Health, 1978), with a clinically reported similarly high rate of breakup among non-marital unions (Williams, 1987). Nor is it surprising that 50 to 80% of women who have been raped report that their marital and/or non-marital relationships ended following the rape (Crenshaw, 1978).

In both distal and proximal STS, the couple's emotional connections and the need to understand the traumatized spouse's ordeal influence the experience of the secondarily affected spouse. The following sections depict, in greater detail, the nature of these effects.

Spouses and Distal Secondary Traumatic Stress

The underlying themes of distal STS are powerlessness and uncertainty. Unable to reach their partners, spouses express a need to know and understand what their partners are going through and whether or not the partner is alive and safe. In an effort to understand what the spouse is going through, the secondarily affected partner may conjure up images of what the missing spouse is going through, based on the available, limited, and possibly incorrect information he or she is able to obtain. Yet, information is often incomplete or contradictory, leading to intense feelings of stress on the part of the secondarily affected spouse. Interestingly, Figley and McCubbin (1983) found that families of American hostages experienced more stress than many of the hostages, primarily because the families had no sense of stability and order, received confusing and contradictory information, and were exposed to new situations that were neither welcomed nor anticipated.

A similar pattern of mis- or disinformation has been seen in families of service persons at the war front. Solomon (1988) has described how technological advancements, particularly television, may introduce information of the most frightening kind into the lives of family members, yet the family has no direct communication with the service person and usually does not know where she or he is. If information is incomplete, spouses will draw on information from other sources. Wives of men serving in "Operation Just Cause" in Panama combined what they knew about the Vietnam War with media accounts of the activities in Panama. The result for these women was heightened anxiety and depression, accompanied, in some cases, by recurring nightmares about their spouses being seriously injured or killed (Scurfield and Tice, 1992). The anxiety and uncertainty are accompanied by role and interactional changes among family members (Solomon, 1988). As a result, stress levels often increase dramatically. Wives of prisoners of war also have been seen to experience this pattern of confusion and uncertainty coupled with a demand to modify role expectations within the family (Ursano and Rundell, 1990).

Wexler and McGrath (1991), in a study of wives' response to husbands' involvement in the Persian Gulf War, found that the majority of respondents reported loneliness, anxiety, sadness, and worry. In addition, a significant minority reported such somatic complaints as headaches, reduced interest in eating, insomnia, feeling distracted, and nervousness. When white women were compared with minority women, the most common negative feeling among white women was anxiety. White women were also more likely to report insomnia and feeling distracted. Minority women, although also anxious, were far more likely than the white women to focus their concern on the welfare of their children.

The pattern of coping with the uncertainty of distal STS is similar to that seen with complicated grief (Rando, 1992). This can be seen in the families of homicide victims discussed by Masters, Friedman, and Getzel (1988). In a study of Vietnam prisoner of war veterans and their wives, Hunter (1978) found that both the wives and their captive husbands exhibited a similar pattern of adjustment to the husband's capture. They described psychological shock and numbing, followed by a period of hyperalertness and attention to detail, followed by a lengthy period of depression, ending in a strong desire (not always acted on) to "move on."

Another relationship between grief and distal STS is that the spouse may be seen by others as attempting to "hold onto something that can never be" or a lack of willingness to "accept reality." Rather than close the family's boundaries and reorganize around the absence of the missing spouse, these individuals maintain the belief that the absent spouse will return. For spouses of men missing in action, past hoaxes and current arguments about the legitimacy of information contributes greatly to the women's anxiety and fears for the safety and whereabouts of their husbands (Morganthau, 1991).

In other MIA cases, wives may have initially grieved what they believed to be their spouses' death, but later came to believe they were not dead and must be located and returned home to their families. Anxiety, fear, frustration, anger, and guilt at initially abandoning the spouse are among the emotions described (Hutchinson, 1992; Mason, 1991).

Although a majority of the literature focuses on war separation and its impact on wives, other examples of situations in which a spouse could experience distal STS might include having a spouse incarcerated in a prison many miles, sometimes several states, away or having a spouse who is receiving medical treatment for a serious or life-threatening condition at a distant location (Halm, 1990; Scurfield & Tice, 1992).

Distal STS may be complicated by the fact that the spouse experiencing distal STS also may be experiencing his or her own PTSD. Arredondo, Orjuela, and Moore (1989) described a case in which a woman illegally immigrated from El Salvador with her three children, leaving her husband behind. She experienced the effects of her own traumas as well as the anxiety tied to the fate of her husband, whom she had been unable to contact.

The impact of distal STS, then, is dependent on a number of factors: the duration of the separation, feelings of helplessness, the degree of uncertainty and danger surrounding the fate of the spouse, the amount and trustworthiness of available information, and one's own experiences. If the missing spouse returns, distal STS may affect the couple's continuing relationship and will likely influence any proximal STS that occurs.

The Spouse and Proximal Secondary Traumatic Stress

Supporting a person who has gone through a traumatic experience can have a powerful and disturbing effect on the person attempting to provide that support, and this may be particularly difficult for a spouse (Ford et al., 1993). Exposure to one's spouse as he or she exhibits symptoms of PTSD may tax and overwhelm the resources of the other spouse. The partner who experienced the traumatic event may be unwilling to discuss it with his or her spouse, while also behaving in an erratic and disruptive fashion. The supportive spouse may then be exposed to the symptoms of PTSD without understanding their cause (Rueger, 1983). The end result could be a disrupted couple relationship with a spouse who attempted to be supportive but was psychologically overwhelmed instead.

Kulka et al. (1990) reported on a national study of Vietnam veterans and their partners (both married and cohabiting) and found that partners of male Vietnam veterans with PTSD had more problems than partners of Vietnam veterans without PTSD. Partners of PTSD-affected veterans reported being less happy and satisfied and having more general distress, including feeling as if they might have a nervous breakdown. They also reported greater social isolation and more family violence. Thus, spouses may experience both the secondary effects of attempting to support a spouse along with the primary effects of their own violent victimization.

In the same study, Kulka et al. also attempted to assess the effects of PTSD on the male partners of female veterans of the war. Unfortunately, due to small sample size, few significant differences were found that differentiated spouses of PTSD-affected female veterans from spouses of non-PTSD-affected female veterans. The spouses of the PTSD-affected female veterans did report lower levels of self-esteem and, curiously, lower levels of social isolation. Although not significant, higher levels of family violence were reported by partners of PTSD-affected female veterans.

In a qualitative study by Maloney (1988), six female partners of Vietnam veterans reported that their panic episodes were set off by triggers similar to their husbands', such as "the sound of helicopters, sudden noises, gunfire, the smell and sound of spring rain, the sight of fog, meeting Oriental people, and the smell of thick humidity" (p. 138). They also spoke of dreaming of Vietnam. As in other studies, their relationships with their spouses were characterized by diminished intimacy.

Patience Mason (1990) drew on her own experience and that of other Vietnam veterans' wives to describe the following long-term symptoms of wives of PTSD-affected Vietnam veterans: rage, at their husbands or at the military; somatic complaints, such as backaches and headaches; distrust of others; hyperalertness, especially for anything that might upset their husbands; depression and thoughts of suicide; feelings of being overwhelmed by the task; numbness; and guilt. She also noted that these women found it difficult to sleep. When they did sleep, they had nightmares in which they dreamt of being in Vietnam or of horrible, uncontrollable things happening to family members, especially their children.

Matsakis (1988) saw similar patterns in women in her spouse support groups. She identified women in her groups who believed they were themselves experiencing symptoms of PTSD, which included insomnia, being easily startled, and dreaming of being in Vietnam. These wives of veterans felt isolated, helpless, and were hypervigilant around their potentially violent husbands, especially with regard to protecting their children. She also reported that, because of societal attitudes toward African-Americans and Hispanics, these women have had an especially difficult time coping, not only with their husbands' PTSD (often made worse by racist attitudes these men experienced on their return to the United States) but with the racism and sexism experienced by these women themselves.

In their support groups for women partners of Vietnam veterans, Coughlan and Parkin (1987) noted that the women seemed to mimic the PTSD symptoms of their husbands. This has also been reported by other scholars who have found that wives of Vietnam veterans diagnosed with PTSD exhibit symptoms similar to their husbands', which included flashbacks and nightmares. These symptoms exacerbate wives' other problems and prevent them from resolving their own stress reactions or providing support to their husbands (Kuenning, 1991; Verbosky & Ryan, 1988; Williams, 1980). Solomon (1988) also found that, following the return of an Israeli soldier/spouse from the front, there are problems with reintegration and erratic behavior of the spouse, resulting in added stress for the other partner and reduced ability on the part of that spouse to be supportive.

Secondary traumatic stress reactions are likely present in other situations that are not war related and are most likely present, in some form, in male partners of female primary victims. Although the bulk of research done on STS has been done on wives of Vietnam veterans, clinicians are aware that it extends to other groups. For instance, Erickson (1989) has suggested that family members of rape victims, including spouses, should be assessed for symptoms of STS.

Mio and Foster's (1991) review of the literature on the effects of rape on victims and families found evidence of proximal STS in spouses and children of rape victims. They described husbands' responses as including rage, frustration, shame, helplessness, guilt, and denial. As with the wives of war veterans, these husbands felt that one of their responsibilities was to protect their wives. This was complicated by their own sense of violation and anger, which, curiously, often was directed toward their wives.

Silverman (1978) suggested that spouses, as well as other family members, may experience the same feelings of helplessness, shock, rage, and physical revulsion felt by the rape victim. They may respond by trying to make decisions for the rape victim, adding to the sense of helplessness of the victim.

Because of the sexual nature of the assault, often compounded by a tendency to "blame the victim," spouses of rape victims may not be able to see beyond the need to locate blame for the rape. Often, this blame is placed on the victim herself (Hertz & Lerer, 1981). The need to question basic assumptions about sexuality and the character of their partner may be too much for many men. As stated earlier in this chapter, the divorce rate is very high for this group.* Miller, Williams, and Bernstein (1982) also found evidence of an impaired relationship when a female partner has been raped, with problems in understanding, commitment, and emotional support; poor communication; and concerns, fears, dissatisfaction, and dysfunction. This group also exhibited a lack of trust, excessive dependency, and a general avoidance of discussion of the rape. If the couple is to recover from the rape, and to remain together as a couple, both partners must deal with their own beliefs and assumptions about rape, themselves, and their relationship. They must also work to correct communication problems they may have.

According to Remer and Elliott (1987a), following a rape, the couple's normal patterns of interaction are impaired. The husband may feel a loss of control and predictability. He may have seen his wife as the nurturer in the family and must now act that role for her, yet, at the same time, he may expect her to nurture him in his crisis (Remer & Elliott, 1987b).

Agosta and McHugh (1987) note that a rape victim's post-rape behavior may lead to confusion and resentment on the part of the supporting spouse. If the victim is ambivalent about or repulsed by the sex act, her spouse may feel angry and rejected. He is also likely to experience helplessness and sadness. In his efforts to come to terms with the rape, he may decide that he was responsible for the rape occurring and may feel a need to control the behavior of his partner.

The timing of the spouse's learning of the rape is also an important factor in dyadic recovery. If there is a long lag time between the occurrence of the rape and when the husband learns of it, the spouses will be at extremely different points in their recovery process and will be dealing with different issues. Remer and Elliott (1987b) suggest that the greater the partners are out of synchrony in their recovery, the more recovery is impaired for both of them. If the victimization took place in the wife's childhood, it would lead to an even more complicated situation for the couple.

---

* I am reminded of a pair of researchers with whom I spoke several years ago about a project they hoped to carry out together. She would interview female victims of rape and he would interview male partners. After several months, they discontinued their efforts to interview the partners, as they were unable to find any women whose partners stayed with them after the rape.

Other examples of proximal STS can be found in the literature. A study was conducted on the aftereffects of a non-fatal military aircraft accident on crew members and squadron members plus the wives of both groups. The spouses were more affected by the accident than crew or squadron members. Of particular note, the wives exhibited higher levels of intrusive thoughts, dreams about the accident, emotional numbing, difficulty in concentrating, feeling emotionally isolated, insomnia, depersonalization, and guilt. Although a small sample (18 servicemen and 10 wives), the findings are intriguing (Slage, Reichman, Rodenhauser, Knoedler & Davis, 1990).

In a long-term study in the Netherlands, which looked at the effect on individuals of being hijacking hostages as well as the effect on members of their families (van der Ploeg & Kleijn, 1989), half of the sample (19% of which were spouses) reported some type of long-term psychological or psychosomatic aftereffect. Specifically, while 46% of the hostages reported longer-lasting avoidance behaviors or phobias, 29% of the family members did as well. Unfortunately, spouses were not separated out from other family members in the analysis, so it is impossible to know which proportion of this affected group was spouses.

In a discussion of the aftermath of criminal victimization, Davis and Friedman (1985) found that persons (who included an unnamed number of spouses)* who attempted to act as supporters to a crime victim had a heightened fear of crime, a feeling of discomfort at listening to the victim tell about the incident, an increase in their own sense of vulnerability, a concern for the victim's safety, and a sense of anger. They experienced increased fear, were more suspicious than before the victimization, felt less safe, and took added precautions. Supporters who were emotionally close to the victims were more likely to take increased precautions and to feel greater fear. They were also more likely to report frequently discussing problems which had resulted from the victimization.

As stated above, most of the research to date has concentrated on wives of returned Vietnam veterans and, to a lesser extent, husbands of rape victims. Proximal STS certainly occurs in other situations. For instance, spouses might experience proximal STS when a partner is

---

* Although specific information on spouses who acted as supporters was not available, in a related report (Friedman, Bischoff, Davis & Person, 1982), the authors indicated that two-thirds of the criminal victims were married; thus, one could assume, with relative comfort, that at least some of the spouses experienced some level of proximal STS.

seriously injured or disabled in an accident yet they also may be placed in the role of "passive participant," wanting to help but unable to do so (Hegeman, 1988). Following the initial crisis, they might be required to take on many of the role responsibilities of the injured spouse, to act as principal or sole supporter, and to deal with emotions that arise in response to the situation. If the injured spouse also suffered a head trauma, the secondarily affected spouse could be in a situation in which he or she has to cope with personality and cognitive deficits of the injured spouse.

In many ways, and to varying degrees, distal STS is influenced by the same factors as proximal STS. Feelings of helplessness and uncertainty characterize both forms. Proximal STS also is characterized by the quality and amount of communication and the nature of interaction with the PTS-affected spouse. Trustworthiness of information is an issue for proximal STS victims, but it may be the primarily affected spouse who is providing untrustworthy data. In addition, proximal STS-affected spouses may be viewed as the principal or only source of support for their partners. Yet, their own needs may be ignored or minimized, leading them to be less supportive. Clearly, the processes of resolving both the primary and secondary traumatic stress are intertwined, and both parties influence each other in their resolution process.

In addition to the secondary traumatization developed in the role of supporter to a spouse, secondary traumatization can also take place in spousal dyads when *both* experience a type of resonating STS. Such exposure might occur when a child becomes suddenly ill, is raped, or is seriously injured. It may also occur when one or both is a primary victim but find their trauma responses triggered by the spouse's actions rather than their own primary traumatization.

RESONATING SECONDARY TRAUMATIC STRESS— WHEN SPOUSES ARE BOTH SECONDARY TRAUMATIC STRESS VICTIMS

Spouses also may experience STS in the context of a couple when they are *both* secondarily affected by someone who is mutually significant to each of them. Placed in a position of trying to understand and provide support to someone important to both partners, they may find that, instead of being able to "lean on one another," they add to the stress felt by each other.

Spouses and Resonating Secondary Traumatic Stress

In an effort to understand and provide support, a couple may experience resonating STS after someone, such as their child, is directly impacted by a traumatic event. In a process similar to what Cornwell, Nurcombe, and Stevens (1977) labeled "resonating grief," the partners would be affected independently of each other, yet, at the same time, their behavior would act as a trigger for each spouse, "setting the other off." Cornwell and his colleagues (Cornwell, Nurcombe & Stevens, 1977) described a pattern of dyadic grieving in which one of the parents would express strong emotions, such as weeping, and the other would respond in a similar fashion. Likewise, partners who experience resonating STS would be triggered by the behavior of their spouses.

Resonating STS among parents has been seen in cases of seriously handicapped children. In one case, a child's health was increasingly fragile, which had contributed to tremendous strain on the parents' relationship. Each time this child experienced a symptom, regardless of whether it was contagious or not, the parents exhibited similar symptoms, always first in the father and then in the mother. On one occasion, the child suffered a head injury while playing and was rendered blind. During recovery, she then had a stroke which paralyzed one side of her body. Within two weeks, her father lost sight in one eye; shortly thereafter, the mother lost feeling on one side of her face. A distinctive characteristic of this couple, according to their daughter's teacher, was that they were both actively invested in their child's welfare and continued to work to keep their lines of communication open with each other (P. Frohliger, personal communication, 1992).

Secondary traumatic stress in a couple context also has been seen in cases of a daughter's rape (Hertz & Lerer, 1981). The marital relationship of the parents can be placed under a great deal of strain as each partner deals with his or her own STS symptoms as well as those of the spouse. A husband might blame his wife for the daughter's problems and may become impotent. He may accuse his daughter of causing or contributing to the rape. The wife may dream of being raped herself and feel resentment toward her husband for his lack of support. She may also accuse the daughter of complicity in her rape. Each person may look for support from others while feeling unable to support anyone himself or herself. Isolation, avoidance, and denial of the seriousness of the situation could contribute to increased tension.

In other cases, only one spouse may exhibit symptoms of STS while the other appears to be quite calm and reserved. In my work with couples who had experienced the death of a child, I often found that men are more likely to focus on the need for emotional control and to deny any anxiety, concentrating more on the need to manage their wives' grief. Wives were more likely to discuss their emotional reaction to their loss and to express concern about their husbands' lack of expressiveness. Men were, however, more likely to exhibit more paralinguistic and body language cues of anxiety (e.g., stuttering, shaking voice, pacing, repeated and rapid crossing of legs), which may be more easily missed when assessing level of anxiety.

It appears, then, from the literature reviewed here that spouses experience secondary effects related either to their partners' direct exposure to a traumatic event or as a sort of "resonating stress" as they must attempt to cope with both their own secondary traumatic stress and that of their partner. But why? What might explain STS among spouses?

THE PROCESS OF SECONDARY TRAUMATIC STRESS IN SPOUSES

There appear to be two principal reasons for the development of STS in spouses. The first centers around a need for stability, understanding, and purpose in their own lives, which incorporates a stable and meaningful relationship with the spouse. The second centers around their emotional connection to the spouse and their desire to help the spouse cope with and resolve (or escape from) the effects of the traumatic stressor. In order to help, however, both partners must first understand what has happened, what it means for each of them, and what it portends for the future. In order to do so as a couple, they must also understand what it means for their partner and their relationship. Ultimately, a shared knowledge base and the ability to support each other are inextricably entwined.

Making Sense of the Traumatic Experience and Its Aftermath

Human beings construct their own personal realities which are made up of "...assumptions, beliefs and expectations about self and world that enable individuals to make sense of their experience" (McCann & Pearlman, 1990, p. 137). Janoff-Bulman (1985, 1992) has proposed that the experience of traumatic stress results in the assault of three basic assumptions shared by most people. Her studies have shown that these include a belief in personal invulnerability, a perception of the world as meaningful and orderly, and a positive view of oneself.

Although Janoff-Bulman refers to direct traumatization when discussing these assumptions and the effects of trauma, as the previously reviewed literature attests, a similar process goes on for STS-affected spouses. With the traumatic experience of a husband or wife, they learn that one is vulnerable, that the world can be meaningless and chaotic, and that being a good person does not protect one from harm.

Rosenthal, Sadler, and Edwards (1987) have noted that these assumptions are shared within families, and when one family member is directly impacted by a trauma, all family members' beliefs are affected. My own research on couples coping with a mutually shared traumatic event (i.e., the death of a baby) confirms that these assumptions about order, predictability, fairness, and protection are extended to one's spouse. Additionally, relational as well as personal assumptions are affected by the trauma (Gilbert & Smart, 1992). Partners may find that, in trying to make sense of a spouse's experience, interactional patterns that facilitated their relationship in the past no longer work for the couple. Yet, stable, trustworthy assumptions are essential for normal life. If the couple is to maintain their relationship as secure, predictable, and meaningful, assumptions must be considered for *both* themselves and their spouse.

Since such an occurrence affects dyadic interactions, when basic beliefs about life are called into question for secondarily affected spouses *or* for their partners, the partners' personal assumptive worlds will be destabilized. The same is true for assumptions about their relationship and related role behavior. Men whose wives have been raped report having difficulty with their wives' inability to act the role of nurturer (Remer & Elliott, 1987a). Women may be confronted with husbands who went to war as kind and gentle men and have returned moody and unstable. In both cases, these spouses must somehow reconcile these changes with their previously held assumptive world. Their own sense of stability has been affected, even though they were not directly traumatized. Spouses do not need to wait for their sense of stability affected. Solomon (1988) found that anticipating these changes (in the case of distal STS) can also affect a spouse's sense of stability.

In order to regain a sense of stability, each partner must attribute meaning and create some sort of explanation, a personal or "healing" theory that will allow him or her to adapt to the changed reality (Figley,

1983, 1985; Taylor, Lichtman & Wood, 1987). Such a healing theory would serve as an explanation for the primary victim's traumatic experience and resultant behavior and the response of the secondarily affected spouse, and a projection into the future to explain forthcoming behavior. Each partner must develop a personal healing theory, and for it to be mutually productive, there must be overlap and the theories must facilitate positive interaction between partners. These will likely be affected by many things. Carroll, Foy, Cannon, and Zwier (1991) have proposed that the following factors be taken into account when considering the marital effects of trauma, all of which will have an effect on the ability to construct a meaningful, functional dyadic healing theory: the point in the relationship at which the trauma occurred; the nature of the relationship *before* the trauma or, if the trauma preceded the relationship, when the partner learned of the trauma; the history of each individual (e.g., other traumas each or both might have experienced, the nature of each person's coping skills, role expectations in the family of origin, etc.); and the severity of impact on each individual and on the relationship.

For spouses dealing with proximal STS or resonating STS, the often unpredictable or unexplainable behavior of the partner may impede the process of theory development (Williams, 1980). The uncertainty regarding the fate of the spouse along with the lack of trustworthiness of information can have the same effect in distal STS. This, then, adds to the stress of the spouse because one way in which one's perceptions are tested and confirmed is through interaction with one's spouse (Berger & Kellner, 1964, 1992). Israelstam (1989) has proposed that the couples establish interacting individual belief systems that influence their cognitive, affective, behavioral, and physiological responses to stress. If one changes, the other changes.

In this model, partners are interconnected and interdependent. One way in which they influence each other is in the construction of a revised reality after a trauma. They are able to consider and validate each other's view of what has happened, is happening, and will happen (Berger & Kellner, 1964, 1992; Reiss, 1981). If their subjective views are confirmed, these views are given objective reality (i.e., what they perceive comes to be seen as reality because significant others also see it that way) (Berger & Luckman, 1966; Holzner, 1968); if not, they question their own or the other's perceptions, and formation of an objective reality is made more difficult (Jay, 1991). If a partner does not get direct feedback from a spouse, he or she may resort to interpretation of the spouse's behavior, which may lead to greater confusion (Israelstam, 1989). Wives of Vietnam veterans have spoken of their self-doubts when they see their husbands as having problems but the husbands deny seeing any (Mason, 1990).

The actions of one's spouse may be perceived by the other in a way that is inconsistent with the intent of the original spouse. For example, in a resonating STS situation, a husband might avoid showing strong emotion in order to help his wife "move on." Rather than seeing this as helpful, she might see it as evidence of his cold and uncaring nature, resulting in avoidance and isolation (Gilbert & Smart, 1992).

Another situation may occur if the primary victim talks about his or her experience. In an effort to process the information and enlighten, others may overwhelm the emotional system of the spouse. The result for the spouse is affect overload, leading to greater susceptibility to STSD (McCann & Pearlman, 1990).

The Couple's Emotional Connection

Following a traumatic experience, the spouse serves the important position of moderating the expression of PTSD in the primary victim (Jones & Barlow, 1990). According to Figley (1986), the functions of the family (and, by extension, the spouse) are to detect symptoms in the primary victim, confront the problem, recapitulate the catastrophe, and resolve trauma-related conflicts. In order to do this, the supporting spouse must gather information about what took place, the effects on the victimized spouse, and *the emotional impact* on the spouse. Because the spousal relationship is an already emotionally charged relationship, these efforts to "connect emotionally" with the spouse's feelings of being out of control, helpless, and caught off guard (Figley, 1989) open the supportive spouse up to the dangers of STS. Thus, it is not so much the images themselves as the underlying affective connection between partners that causes STS.

In order to understand the traumatic stress experience (whether PTS or STS) of a spouse and know when and how to help him or her, the supportive spouse must "borrow" the images and memories of her or his partner. McCann and Pearlman (1990) described the secondary traumatization of therapists who attempted to empathize with PTSD clients by taking on their memories. This allowed them to better serve their clients but put them at risk of losing the "as if" quality to their images and taking on the memories as their own. They suggested that therapists retain emotional distance in order to protect themselves from these memories. Corcoran (1989) made a similar suggestion to avoid burnout.

For spouses, this maintenance of emotional distance is generally not possible. Marital partners are seen as interdependent, emotionally and communicationally (Levinger & Huston, 1990). To emotionally disengage is not a socially approved method of coping with one another's distress (Blood & Wolfe, 1960; Burke & Weir, 1977). According to Blumstein and Schwartz (1983), "Two people become a couple in large measure to secure a trustworthy source of affection—emotional as well as physical" (p. 194). Compounding this assumption of affective closeness is an assumption of continuity in the relationship, a factor which Blumstein and Schwartz found to be true for both marital and nonmarital relationships. Thus, the added sense of commitment and love in some cases, and fear and a sense of inescapable danger in others, compounds the likelihood of spouses developing STSR or STSD.

In an effort to support and empathize with the troubled spouse, the person who is attempting to be supportive often takes on the other's images and memories as his or her own. The end result, as indicated in the literature reviewed previously, is that the supportive spouse indirectly experiences the primarily victimized spouse's trauma. A secondarily affected spouse who is overwhelmed by these borrowed memories may then avoid his or her spouse, deny the problem, or be emotionally overwhelmed (McCann & Pearlman, 1990). This, compounded by an emotionally numbed PTSD victim, can lead to feelings of alienation between partners (Kuenning, 1991; Rosenchek & Thomson, 1986; Scaturo & Harbody, 1988).

Another aspect of the emotional/intimacy bond of the couple is their sexual relationship. Sexual problems may contribute to the overall strain in the relationship. Veterans returning from war may find their sexual drive diminished, while their wives may feel rejected and unloved (Williams, 1980). Women who spoke with Kuenning (1991) described their Vietnam veteran husbands as either too demanding or disinterested. Others have noted a similar change in the sexual relationship of Vietnam vet couples (Mason, 1990; Matsakis, 1988).

The situation involving rape is even more complicated because, aside from everything else, the spouse also must come to terms with his own ideas about sexuality, exclusivity, and cultural myths about rape as a sexual crime (Mio & Foster, 1991; Remer & Elliott, 1987a).

COMPLICATIONS OF CARING TOO MUCH

Given the expectations of couples, it should be no surprise that when one spouse experiences a trauma, the other feels duty-bound to support his or her spouse. Marital partners are seen as a primary source of social support for their spouses (Blood & Wolfe, 1960; Burke & Weir, 1977). For many couples, one's spouse may be seen as one of several primary sources of support; he or she may be seen as *the only* source of support (Gilbert & Smart, 1992; Orzek, 1983).

Having a PTSD-affected spouse is distressing and disruptive. Yet, spouses who have been placed in a supporting role are not able to focus on their own experience. They also must cope with and respond to their spouses and the spouses' needs. Rather than simply focus on their own experience, supporting spouses must also cope with what they believes the spouse's experience to be. This is done by attempting to anticipate the meaning of the event and its emotional impact on the spouse. This is not completely altruistic, as spouses cast in the supporting role may not receive much support themselves. To reduce their own felt stress (in response to the spouse), they must respond in some way to their spouses' behavior. This may, however, lead to overload on the part of supporting spouses and contribute to their own secondary traumatic stress. As indicated before, spouses exist in an interactive, interdependent system, and if one spouse must continually act the supporter without receiving support in return, that person ultimately may be overwhelmed. Therefore, it is important that both spouses learn to act as supporters for each other (Williams, 1987).

Overresponsibility and Overfunctioning

I was reminded recently, while attending a wedding, of a curious expectation which has been placed on marital partners. The mother of the bride, in toasting the couple, encouraged them to remember that "...once you were two, now you are one." This sentiment is expressed by scholars writing positively of the interdependence of the marital couple (Burke & Weir, 1977, 1982; Rands & Levinger, 1979). Blumstein and Schwartz (1983) have indicated that this sense of interdependence extends to non-marital couples as well.

When a traumatic stressor occurs, this interdependence may move to a less healthy form. Scaturo and Harbody (1988) spoke of "interlocking pathologies" in couples in which one was experiencing PTSD.

Mason (1990) referred to her own behavior and that of other wives of Vietnam veterans as "co-dependent," a situation in which the spouse takes on the responsibility of solving the problems of the PTSD-affected spouse. Scaturo and Harbody (1988) observed this in wives of Vietnam veterans only if they had married after the men returned from Vietnam and suggested that these women may see this as "part of the package" of marrying these men. They also noted that, among the population they served, wives who were married before Vietnam did not stay with their PTSD-affected spouses. Serving a different sample of women in partner support groups, Coughlan and Parkin (1987) did not see any difference in the wives whether they had been married before or after their husbands went to Vietnam. What they and others serving spouses of Vietnam veterans saw was a mixture of a sense of responsibility toward their spouses, their children, others, and, in many instances, themselves. Guilt, low self-esteem, and fear also were powerful motivators for their taking on the role of "the responsible one" (Mason, 1990) or "the nurturing one" (Solomon, 1988) in the family. The result is a sense of being overwhelmed by the constant barrage of demands placed on them.

Similarly, male partners of rape victims may feel a sense of responsibility toward the victim and became hypervigilant in protecting her, sometimes pushing her toward a feeling of powerlessness (Mio & Foster, 1991). The extent to which a man will take on this responsibility is influenced by his education level, degree of commitment to the relationship, willingness to struggle with difficulties, and his own stages of coping (Remer & Elliott, 1987a).

Because women are frequently seen (and see themselves) as the keepers of the home, they are particularly susceptible to taking on most if not all of the responsibility for maintaining the emotional climate in the family (Mason, 1990). Williams (1980) described wives and partners of Vietnam veterans as caught in the "compassion trap." These women have also spoken of "walking on eggshells" (Matsakis, 1988) in an effort to keep from upsetting their husbands. Wives, it appears, are caught in the role of helper to their husbands as these men cope with their PTSD (Mason, 1990; Scaturo & Harbody, 1988).

By overfunctioning, the woman not only increases her own stress but also adds to the disenfranchisement of her husband from the family. Her efforts to fulfill roles traditionally held by the husband may be seen by him as evidence that she believes him to be incapable of carrying out his role (Bleich, Garb & Kottler, 1986; Solomon, 1988). Alternatively, he may also contribute to his own disenfranchisement by abandoning those roles when he sees her as willing to take them on (DeFazio & Pascucci, 1984).

If there are children in the family, the wife may attempt to protect them from the perceived or real threat of the spouse (Mason, 1990; Matsakis, 1988). In addition, she may also try to help her children understand the erratic behavior of the PTSD-affected partner. In either case, her efforts to understand and explain her husband's behavior will add to her own stress.

Guilt may be the motivating force behind her efforts to compensate for her spouse (Verbosky & Ryan, 1988). She may feel helpless to change him and he may identify her as the cause of the problems. This may also contribute to increased animosity, reduced supportiveness, or even the disintegration of the marriage.

Overprotection and Spousal Isolation

Because of the obvious difficulties inherent in discussions of the trauma and its aftereffects, spouses may attempt to avoid situations in which these are addressed. Mason (1990) described her acting out the role of enabler of her husband's PTSD by attempting to protect him and adjust to him without actually helping him to deal with his troubling memories. She found that other vets' wives did the same thing.

Primary victims may isolate themselves from others, including the spouse, because it is too painful to talk about the event. They may have attempted to do so in the past, and if their spouses responded with shock or dismay, they might have been unable to accept the perceived rejection. On the other hand, the secondary victim may be tired of hearing about the event or may find it uncomfortable to perceive the spouse as vulnerable. The partner may then have urged the primary victim to "put it behind you" and "get on with your life," also affecting the willingness of the spouse to share (Gilbert & Smart, 1992).

Whatever the motivation, this overprotectiveness diminishes their ability to communicate with each other. Yet, effective communication is essential to successful dyadic functioning (Epstein & Westley, 1959; Figley, 1983). Therefore, by avoiding interacting with each other, both partners may end up feeling isolated and without support.

If spouses are unable to test and confirm their reality with the PTSD-affected spouse, they may look to others to do this. But support is often not forthcoming. Couples in which one partner suffers from the effects of PTSD are often socially isolated. The drive to isolate the family may come from inside or from outside the family. The PTSD-affected spouse may be instrumental in preventing family members from seeing others (Glassman, Magulac & Darko, 1987; Maloney, 1988). STS-affected spouses may feel that others cannot understand what they are going through. The outside social network may not want to hear about their problems. Mason (1990) found that when she sought support from her extended family and friends, they responded with, "Why do you stay with him?"

Spouses may not be seen as entitled to support from others. As indicated earlier, they may be seen as having primary responsibility for providing support to the PTSD victim—there to provide support, not be supported. In addition, spouses affected indirectly by the trauma may feel that they lack legitimacy in seeking support from others. It may be that they see their spouse's support needs as more important than their own. The paucity of available support or a self-perception of weakness ("I was not be able to help my partner.") may keep them from getting the help that they need, which adds to their feeling of being over-whelmed and alone.

Marital Distress and Spousal Violence

When one partner has PTSD, the demands placed on the other partner are extremely high. As Kulka et al. (1990) found, spousal relationships are highly disrupted when one partner has PTSD. Spousal violence or the threat of violence toward the spouse of a PTSD victim often is present in such relationships (Verbosky & Ryan, 1988; Kulka et al., 1990; Kuenning, 1991; Mason, 1990). Drug and alcohol abuse in one or both partners are also potential problems, as are other addictive or compulsive behaviors (Mason, 1990).

A common report in individual therapy and support groups for wives and female partners is that these women must cope with a highly unpredictable husband who may threaten or become violent. They may, therefore, suffer STS effects from their efforts to empathize with their husbands' traumatic experiences while also experiencing their own PTSD which is related to spousal violence (Maloney, 1988).

IMPLICATIONS FOR INTERVENTION IN THE CONTEXT OF SPOUSES

In this section, intervention with couples will be briefly addressed. A detailed description of a treatment approach for producing secondary survivors of traumatic stress is available elsewhere in this volume.

When one partner experiences a traumatic stressor, a safe assumption is that the other also suffers. In order to maintain his or her own sense of stability and meaning, as well as the stability of the dyadic relationship, the spouse must attempt to make sense of his or her partner's experience and the impact that it has on their lives together. This, coupled with the emotional connection between the partners, exposes the spouse to the risks of STS. This can occur whether the spouses are separated or in continued contact after the trauma, and in both conditions, the underlying issues are a need to care for the affected spouse and the uncertainty of what has happened, is happening, and will happen.

Therapeutic intervention with this population may be difficult to initiate. Because spouses may be unwilling or unable to seek help, care providers should seek them out (Solomon, 1988). Male partners of rape victims, for example, may need help in recognizing their feelings about the rape and learning to express them in healthy ways (Agosta & McHugh, 1987). Female partners, in general, may need help in overcoming their socially encouraged tendency to overfunction. Spouses of both genders need to be helped to recognize their obligation to provide support to their secondarily affected spouses.

Figley (1989) has suggested a five-step family therapy treatment program for families coping with traumatic stress that focuses on the following objectives: building rapport and trust between the therapist and the client family, clarifying the therapist's role, eliminating unwanted consequences of the traumatic experience, building family social supportiveness, developing new rules and skills for family communication, promoting self-disclosure, recapitulating the traumatic event, and building a family healing theory. Using such an approach would build the couple's sense of working together as a team to resolve their stress.

Another family approach, based on the theoretical concepts of Viktor Frankl, includes five stages: establishing the treatment system, remembering terror, recovering meaning in trauma and terror, making use of meaning potentials, and termination and celebration. This intervention includes the entire family, and family members work together as a group in resolving their traumatized condition (Lantz & Lantz, 1991).

In order for the couple to move toward healthy functioning as a marital unit, marital therapy will be a necessary component of intervention (Solomon, Waysman, Avitzur & Enoch, 1991). According to Carroll et al. (1991), the areas of marital functioning most affected by trauma are expressiveness, intimacy, and overt hostility. Couple communication and the sexual relationship are also important treatment issues. Another use for marital therapy is that it will allow a couple whose recovery is out of synchrony (i.e., they are at radically different points in their recovery) to synchronize their movement toward resolution (Remer & Elliott, 1987b).

Others have suggested individual therapy for partners, so that they can work on their own issues. Williams (1980) has suggested that before doing any type of couple therapy, each spouse should receive individual therapy, with the wife's therapy focusing on increasing assertiveness and recognizing her own needs, a view shared by Solomon (1988). Matsakis (1988) recommends that female partners affected by STS see a feminist or a non-sexist counselor. Rabin and Nardi (1991) suggest a psychoeducational approach in both individual and group formats, as they believe this carries less stigma than a clinical therapeutic model.

Ultimately, it appears that the most appropriate approach to treatment of a couple would be a combination of individual and couple sessions targeted at specific issues (Carroll et al., 1991).

SUMMARY

The ways in which spouses are affected by STS have been explored in this chapter. Spouses may be at particular risk for development of STSR or STSD because of the uniquely close and emotional nature of the spousal relationship. STS may be the result of direct (i.e., proximal) or indirect (i.e., distal) exposure to the primary victimization of one's spouse. In addition, spouses can experience a type of resonating STS reaction in which they trigger each other's STS response.

The STS responses of spouses seem to result from their need to make sense of the traumatic experience and its aftermath while they are also working to maintain a stable and workable relationship with their partner. The end result of this may be that secondarily affected spouses become overresponsible and overfunction for their partners. Efforts to protect the primarily affected spouse may actually result in the overprotection and isolation of the spouse. Therefore, given the nature of the relationship and the need to learn new ways of knowing and new behaviors, the therapeutic plan for these couples should incorporate both individual and couple therapy.

REFERENCES

Agosta, C.A., & McHugh, M.L. (1987). Sexual assault victims: The trauma and the healing. In T. Williams (Ed.), *Post-traumatic stress disorders: A handbook for clinicians* (pp. 239–251). Cincinnati, OH: Disabled American Veterans.

Arredondo, P., Orjuela, E., & Moore, L. (1989). Family therapy with Central American war refugee families. *Journal of Strategic and Systemic Therapies, 8,* 28–35.

Berger, P., & Kellner, H. (1964/1992). Marriage and the construction of reality: An exercise in the microsociology of knowledge. *Diogenes, 46,* 1–25; reprinted in J.M. Henslin (Ed.), *Marriage and family in a changing society* (4th ed.). New York: The Free Press.

Berger, P., & Luckman, T. (1966). *The social construction of reality.* New York: Doubleday.

Bleich, A., Garb, R., & Kottler, M. (1986). Treatment of prolonged combat reaction. *British Journal of Psychiatry, 148,* 493–496.

Blood, R.O., & Wolfe, D.M. (1960). *Husbands and wives: The dynamics of married living.* New York: The Free Press.

Blumstein, P., & Schwartz, P. (1983). *American couples.* New York: William Morrow and Co.

Boss, P. (1987). Family stress. In M.B. Sussman and S.K. Steinmetz (Eds.), *Handbook of marriage and the family* (pp. 695–724). New York: Plenum Press.

Boss, P. (1991). The other victims: Families of hostages. *USA Today Magazine, 120,* 68–69.

Burke, R.J., & Weir, T. (1977). Marital helping relationships: The moderators between stress and well being. *The Journal of Psychology, 95,* 121–130.

Burke, R.J., & Weir, T. (1982). Husband-wife helping relationships as moderators of experienced stress: The "mental hygiene" function in marriage. In H.I. McCubbin, A.E. Cauble, and J.M. Patterson (Eds.), *Family stress, coping, and social support* (pp. 221–238). Springfield, IL: Charles C Thomas.

Carroll, E.M., Foy, D.W., Cannon, B.J., & Zwier, G. (1991). Assessment issues involving the families of trauma victims. *Journal of Traumatic Stress, 4,* 25–40.

Corcoran, K.J. (1989). Interpersonal stress and burnout: Unraveling the role of empathy. *Journal of Social Behavior and Psychiatry, 4,* 141–144.

Cornwell, J., Nurcombe, B., & Stevens, L. (1977). Family response to the loss of a child by Sudden Infant Death Syndrome. *Medical Journal of Australia, 1,* 656–658.

Coughlan, K., & Parkin, C. (1987). Women partners of Vietnam vets. *Journal of Psychosocial Nursing, 25*(10), 25–27.

Crenshaw, T.L. (1978). Counseling the family and friends. In S. Halper (Ed.), *Rape: Helping the victim* (pp. 51–65). Oredell, NJ: Medical Economics Book Division.

Davis, R.C., & Friedman, L.N. (1985). The emotional aftermath of crime and violence. In C. Figley (Ed.), *Trauma and its wake, Volume I: The study and treatment of post-traumatic stress disorder* (pp. 90–112). New York: Brunner/Mazel.

DeFazio, V.J., & Pascucci, N.J. (1984). Return to Ithaca: A perspective on marriage and love in post traumatic stress disorder. *Journal of Contemporary Psychotherapy, 14,* 76–89.

Epstein, N., & Westley, W. (1959). Patterns of intrafamilial communication. *Psychiatric Research Reports, 11,* 1–12.

Erickson, C.A. (1989). Rape and the family. In C.R. Figley (Ed.), *Treating stress in families* (pp. 257–290). New York: Brunner/Mazel.

Figley, C.R. (1983). Catastrophes: An overview of family reactions. In C.R. Figley and H.I. McCubbin (Eds.), *Stress and the family, Volume II: Coping with catastrophe* (pp. 3–20). New York: Brunner/Mazel.

Figley, C.R. (1985). From victim to survivor: Social responsibility in the wake of a catastrophe. In C.R. Figley (Ed.), *Trauma and its wake, Volume I: The study and treatment of post-traumatic stress disorder* (pp. 398–413). New York: Brunner/Mazel.

Figley, C.R. (1986). Traumatic stress: The role of the family and social support system. In C.R. Figley (Ed.), *Trauma and its wake, Volume II: Traumatic stress, theory, research, and intervention* (pp. 39–54). New York: Brunner/Mazel.

Figley, C.R. (1989). *Helping traumatized families,* San Francisco: Jossey-Bass.

Figley, C.R. (1995). *Compassion fatigue: Coping with secondary traumatic stress disorder in those who treat the traumatized.* New York: Brunner/Mazel.

Figley, C.R., & McCubbin, H.I. (Eds.) (1983). *Stress and the family, Volume II: Coping with catastrophe.* New York: Brunner/Mazel.

Ford, J.D., Shaw, D., Sennhauser, S., Greaves, D., Thacker, B., Chandler, P., Schwartz, L., & McClain, V. (1993). Psychosocial debriefing after Operation Desert Storm: Marital and family assessment and intervention. *Journal of Social Issues, 49,* 73–102.

Friedman, K., Bischoff, H., Davis, R.C., & Person, A. (1982). *Victims and Helpers: Reactions to Crime.* New York: Victim Services Agency.

Gilbert, K.R., & Smart, L.S. (1992). *Coping with infant or fetal loss: The couple's healing process.* New York: Brunner/Mazel.

Glassman, J.N.S., Magulac, M., & Darko, D.F. (1987). Folie a famille: Shared paranoid disorder in a Vietnam veteran and his family. *American Journal of Psychiatry, 144*(5), 658–660.

Halm, M.A. (1990). Effects of support groups on anxiety of family members during critical illness. *Heart & Lung, 19,* 62–71.

Hegeman, K.M. (1988). A care plan for the family of a brain trauma client. *Rehabilitation Nursing, 13,* 254–258, 262.

Hertz, D.G., & Lerer, B. (1981). The "rape family": Family reactions to the rape victim. *International Journal of Family Psychiatry, 2*, 301–315.

Holzner, B. (1968). *Reality construction in society.* Cambridge, MA: Schankman Publishing.

Hunter, E.J. (1978). The Vietnam POW veteran: Immediate and long-term effects of captivity. In C.R. Figley (Ed.), *Stress disorders among Vietnam veterans: Theory, research and treatment* (pp. 188–206). New York: Brunner/Mazel.

Hutchinson, J. (1992). Missing in action. *Chicago Tribune*, January 5, 1992, Sect. 6, 3.

Israelstam, K.V. (1989). Interacting individual belief systems in marital relationships. *Journal of Marital and Family Therapy, 15*, 53–63.

Janoff-Bulman, R. (1985). The aftermath of victimization: Rebuilding shattered assumptions. In C.R. Figley (Ed.), *Trauma and its wake: The study and treatment of post-traumatic stress disorder* (pp. 15–35). New York: Brunner/Mazel.

Janoff-Bulman, R. (1992). *Shattered assumptions: Toward a new psychology of trauma.* New York: The Free Press.

Jay, J. (1991). Terrible knowledge. *Family Therapy Networker*, November/December, 19–29.

Jones, J.C., & Barlow, D.H. (1990). The etiology of posttraumatic stress disorder. *Clinical Psychology Review, 10*, 299–328.

Kuenning, D.A. (1991). *Life after Vietnam: How veterans and their loved ones can heal the psychological wounds of war.* New York: Paragon Press.

Kulka, R.A., Schlenger, W.E., Fairbank, J.A., Hough, R.L., Jordan, B.K., Marmar, C.R., & Weiss, D.S. (1990). *Trauma and the Vietnam War generation: Report of findings from the national Vietnam veterans readjustment study.* New York: Brunner/Mazel.

Lantz, J. & Lantz, J. (1991). Franklian treatment with the traumatized family. *Journal of Family Psychotherapy, 2*, 61–72.

Levinger, G., & Huston, T.L. (1990). The social psychology of marriage, In F.D. Fincham and T.N. Bradbury (Eds.), *The social psychology of marriage* (pp. 19–58). New York: Guilford Press.

Maloney, L.J. (1988). Post traumatic stresses of women partners of Vietnam veterans. *Smith College Studies in Social Work, 58*, 122–143.

Mason, M. (1991). "I say a prayer and push on." *Newsweek, 118,* 26.

Mason, P.H.C. (1990). *Recovering from the war: A woman's guide to helping your Vietnam vet, your family, and yourself.* New York: Penguin Books.

Masters, R., Friedman, L.N., & Getzel, G. (1988). Helping families of homicide victims: A multidimensional approach. *Journal of Traumatic Stress, 1*(1), 109–125.

Matsakis, A. (1988). *Vietnam wives: Women and children surviving life with veterans suffering post traumatic stress disorder.* Kensington, MD: Woodbine House.

McCann, I.L., & Pearlman, L.A. (1990). Vicarious traumatization: A framework for understanding the psychological effects of working with victims. *Journal of Traumatic Stress, 3*, 131–150.

Miller, W.R., Williams, A.M., & Bernstein, M.H. (1982). The effects of rape on marital and sexual adjustment. *American Journal of Family Therapy, 10*, 51–58.

Mio, J.S., & Foster, J.D. (1991). The effects of rape upon victims and families: Implications for a comprehensive family therapy. *American Journal of Family Therapy, 19,* 147–159.

Morganthau, T. (1991). Hoping against hope. *Newsweek, 118,* 20–26.

Orzek, A.M. (1983). Sexual assault: The female victim, her male partner, and their relationship. *The Personnel and Guidance Journal, 62,* 143–146.

President's Commission on Mental Health. (1978). *Mental health problems of Vietnam era veterans, Volume 3* (pp. 1321–1328).

Rabin, C., & Nardi, C. (1991). Treating post traumatic stress disorder couples: A psychoeducational program. *Community Mental Health Journal, 27*(3), 209–224.

Rando, T.A. (1992). The increasing prevalence of complicated mourning: The onslaught is just beginning. *Omega, 26,* 43–59.

Rands, M., & Levinger, G. (1979). Implicit theories of relationship: An intergenerational study. *Journal of Personality and Social Psychology, 37,* 645–661.

Reiss, D. (1981). *The family's construction of reality.* Cambridge, MA: Harvard University Press.

Remer, R., & Elliott, J.E. (1987a). *Characteristics of secondary victims of sexual assault.* Unpublished manuscript.

Remer, R., & Elliott, J.E. (1987b). *Management of secondary victims of sexual assault.* Unpublished manuscript.

Rosenchek, R., & Thomson, J. (1986). "Detoxification" of Vietnam war trauma: A combined family-individual approach. *Family Process, 25,* 559–570.

Rosenthal, D., Sadler, A., & Edwards, W. (1987). Families and post-traumatic stress disorder. *The Family Therapy Collection, 22,* 81–95.

Rueger, D.B. (1983). Posttraumatic stress disorder: Analysis of female partners' relationship perception, Paper presented at the annual meeting of the American Psychological Association, Anaheim, CA; cited in Carroll, E.M., Foy, D.W., Cann, B.J., & Zweir, G. (1991) *Journal of Traumatic Stress, 4,* 25–40.

Scaturo, D.J., & Hardoby, W.J. (1988). Psychotherapy with traumatized Vietnam combatants: An overview of individual, group, and family treatment modalities. *Military Medicine, 153,* 262–269.

Scurfield, R.M., & Tice, S.N. (1992). Intervention with medical and psychiatric evacuees and their families: From Vietnam through the Gulf war. *Military Medicine, 157,* 88–97.

Silverman, D.C. (1978). Sharing the crisis of rape: Counseling the mates and families of victims. *American Journal of Orthopsychiatry, 48,* 166–173.

Slage, D.A., Reichman, M., Rodenhauser, P., Knoedler, D., & Davis, C.L. (1990). Community psychological effects following a non-fatal aircraft accident. *Aviation, Space & Environmental Medicine, 61*(10), 879–886.

Solomon, Z. (1988). The effect of combat-related posttraumatic stress disorder on the family. *Psychiatry, 51,* 323–329.

Solomon, Z., Waysman, M., Avitzur, E., & Enoch, D. (1991). Psychiatric symptomology among wives of soldiers following combat stress reaction: The role of the social network and marital relations. *Anxiety Research, 4,* 213–223.

Taylor, S.E., Lichtman, R.R., & Wood, J.V. (1987). Attribution, beliefs about control and adjustment to breast cancer. *Journal of Personality and Social Psychology, 46,* 489–502.

Terr, L.C. (1989). Family anxiety after traumatic events. *Journal of Clinical Psychiatry, 50,* 15–19.

Ursano, R.J., & Rundell, J.R. (1990). The prisoner of war. *Military Medicine, 155,* 176–180.

van der Ploeg, H.M., & Kleijn, W.C. (1989). Being held hostage in the Netherlands: A study of long-term aftereffects. *Journal of Traumatic Stress, 2,* 153–169.

Verbosky, S.J., & Ryan, D.A. (1988). Female partners of Vietnam veterans: Stress by proximity. *Issues in Mental Health Nursing, 9,* 95–104.

Wexler, H.K., & McGrath, E. (1991). Family member stress reactions to military involvement separation. *Psychotherapy, 28,* 515–519.

Williams, C.M. (1980). The veteran system—With a focus on woman partners: Theoretical considerations, problems and treatment strategies. In T. Williams (Ed.), *Post-traumatic stress disorders of the Vietnam veteran* (pp. 73–117). Cincinnati, OH: Disabled American Veterans.

Williams, C.M. (1987). The veteran system with a focus on woman partners. In T. Williams (Ed.), *Post-traumatic stress disorders: A handbook for clinicians* (pp. 169–192). Cincinnati, OH: Disabled American Veterans.

UNDERSTANDING THE SECONDARY TRAUMATIC STRESS OF PARENTS

4

Michael F. Barnes, Ph.D.

INTRODUCTION

Parents are traumatized when their child has been injured. If you don't believe it, visit a hospital emergency waiting room some time. Our daily news is filled with stories of these sudden, unexpected accidents, injuries, and illnesses that befall the children of even the most cautious parents. Semonin-Holleran (1991) states that approximately 20,000 pediatric patients die each year from traumatic accidents, while another 100,000 are permanently disabled from the improper use of infant cribs or car seats, falls from heights, bicycle and automobile accidents, sports injuries, and gunshot wounds. It is clear from the traumatology literature (Jones & Peterson, 1993; Lipovsky, 1991) that physically abused, severely injured children show signs of psychological trauma.

For the vast majority of these traumatized children, family members are at risk, too. They have either witnessed the traumatizing event or have received notification of their child's injuries. Many of these families are forced to endure long periods of medical or psychological treatment in which possible death or long-term physical, intellectual, and emotional disabilities remain in question.

1-57444-047-0/98/$0.00+$.50
© 1998 by CRC Press LLC

Many families will be forced to live for months or years with chronic physical disabilities and/or emotional scars that their children received from the traumatizing event. While medical and psychological services are available for the traumatized child, the child's family and friends are often excluded from services because they do not fit our definition of trauma victim.

Secondary traumatic stress is defined by Figley (1995) as the "natural consequent behaviors and emotions resulting from knowing about a traumatizing event experienced by a significant other—the stress resulting from helping or wanting to help a traumatized or suffering person" (p. 7). Parents who must deal with the sudden traumatization of someone they love; who must cope with the physical, emotional, and behavioral changes that often follow the trauma; and who must face their own uncertainty and personal vulnerability are clearly candidates for this secondary traumatization.

Fortunately for the parents of traumatized children, a growing number of traumatology scholars recognize that family members and professionals who work with trauma victims appear to experience their own set of symptoms which are remarkably similar to those experienced by the trauma victim. Concepts such as secondary traumatization (Figley, 1983, 1986, 1988, 1989, 1990; Rosenheck & Nathan, 1985), vicarious traumatization (McCann & Pearlman, 1990), chiasmal effects of traumatization (Kisher, 1984), and compassion fatigue (Figley, 1993; 1995) are all references to the process of the systemic traumatization of individuals who come in close, frequent proximity to, and maintain empathy for, victims of traumatic events.

Clearly, the majority of the seminal works in the study of secondary traumatization have focused on the systemic interactional patterns of adult trauma survivors and their family members. These include, for example, such populations as adult survivors of war (Rosenheck, 1986; Rosenheck & Nathan, 1985; Silver & Iacono, 1986), rape (Feinauer, 1982; Mio & Foster, 1991), crime (Kisher, 1984), and the study of medical and mental health professionals who work with traumatized individuals (Figley, 1993; 1995; McCann & Pearlman, 1990).

There is a growing body of theoretical and research literature that has investigated the response patterns and experiences of families of murdered, critically ill, injured, and disabled children. Barnes (1995) reviewed traumatology and other professional literature (i.e., nursing, family medicine, pediatric cancer, and head trauma/rehabilitation) associated with the impact of chronic illness or sudden injury of children on their members. His review indicates that there appear to be significant similarities between the symptoms cited in the child-focused literature and the literature mentioned above concerning adult trauma survivors. The following is a discussion of primary and secondary trauma symptoms, as well as a review of research-based literature associated with the secondary traumatization of families. The chapter concludes with a review of the axioms that have been identified from the literature review and upon which future research questions can be developed.

SECONDARY TRAUMATIC STRESS

Figley (1995) states that while secondary traumatic stress disorder would be experienced by the victim as a syndrome of symptoms that are nearly identical to post-traumatic stress disorder (PTSD), "there is a fundamental difference between the sequelae or pattern of response during and following a traumatic event for those exposed to primary and secondary stressors" (p. 8). The fundamental difference is that the primary trauma victim experiences symptoms that are directly associated with some aspect of the traumatic event, whereas the secondary trauma victim experiences symptoms that are associated with the primary trauma victim.

A REVIEW OF FINDINGS FROM ADULT-BASED LITERATURE

Several authors (Burr, Klein & Associates, 1994; Figley, 1988; McCubbin & McCubbin, 1989; McCubbin & Patterson, 1989) cite Hills's (1949) classic study as the first to focus on the effects of traumatic stress on the family system. While Figley (1992) states that the majority of the traumatology literature has focused on the primary trauma victim, missing those who were indirectly or secondarily traumatized, several research studies have been carried out on the families of adult trauma survivors. The types of traumatization most commonly studied include war, rape, and death by homicide.

War

Of those empirical studies that have addressed the issue of secondary traumatization and the families of adult trauma survivors, the most significant area of study has been the effects of war on the veterans' family systems. The works of Carroll, Rueger, Foy, and Donahoe (1985); Kulka, Schlenger, Fairbanks, Hough, Jordan, Marmar, and Weiss (1990); Silver and Iacono (1986); Solomon, Mikulincer, Freid, and Wosner (1987); and Solomon, Waysman, Levy, Freid, Mikulincer, Benbenishty, Florian, and Bleich (1992) all address the interactional process that results when a marital or relational system adjusts to a member with PTSD. Findings from this research indicate that both the PTSD sufferer and his or her spouse/partner experience difficulty with expressiveness and marital/relationship satisfaction, higher incidence of marital/relationship problems with lower perceived marital/relationship adjustment, and higher reported conflict and hostility. Another set of findings suggests that the PTSD sufferer and his or her spouse/partner may both experience PTSD-like symptoms and that the experience of these symptoms may be prolonged by the interactional/coping patterns that have been developed by each individual to deal with the PTSD symptoms of his or her partner.

Rape

In addition to war, rape-related PTSD causes stress in families. Two resources were found in the traumatology literature that address the family response to rape. Feinauer (1982) and Mio and Foster (1991) agree that family members experience their own traumatization after becoming aware of the rape of a loved one. Many families respond with denial of the traumatic event, which often serves as a covert call for silence about the event and associated symptoms. This denial sends a message to the victim to keep the event a secret, which enables each family member to avoid dealing openly with his or her issues associated with the event.

The functioning of a family system is altered in response to the traumatization of a family member. In their discussion of interactional changes that occur between the father or husband and the rape victim, Feinauer (1992) and Mio and Foster (1991) have found that a pattern of overprotectiveness is often experienced. They view this pattern as a defensive reaction on the part of the male for not being able to defend his loved one and a means of avoiding feelings of anger and rage at the attacker and the victim for forcing him to deal with this painful event. In addition to the points established above, Mio and Foster (1991) propose that the family of the rape victim may experience the same "feelings of helplessness, shock, rage, or physical revulsion that are experienced by the victim" (p. 151).

Death by Homicide

Amick-McMullan, Kilpatrick, Veronen, and Smith (1989) completed an exploratory study on the family response patterns following the homicidal murder of a family member. Results of this study indicate that 68% of the subjects scored sufficiently high on indicators of depression, somatization, anxiety, and phobic anxiety to warrant the need for ongoing assessment and treatment. They also report that 100% of the survivors reported some degree of event-related symptoms, which would be characteristic of PTSD. These PTSD-like symptoms were found to be unrelated to the gender of the subject. Other findings indicate that, like primary trauma victims, the surviving family members will also experience symptoms on cognitive, affective, physiological, and behavioral dimensions. Also, like primary trauma victims, reminders of the homicide were found to elicit aversive intrusive thoughts and feelings, as well as behavioral avoidance of homicide cues in the surviving family members studied.

SECONDARY TRAUMATIZATION OF PARENTS

There are few research articles that address the issues associated with the secondary traumatization of parents and other family members of traumatized children. In fact, a review of the traumatology literature uncovered only three. Applebaum and Burns (1991) completed a quantitative study on the occurrence of PTSD symptoms in siblings and parents of children who died sudden, unexpected deaths. The findings indicate that both siblings (45%) and parents (35%) of children who are suddenly killed report symptoms that would be consistent with the diagnosis of PTSD.

It is interesting to note that a high correlation was not found between a child's self-report of PTSD symptoms and his or her parents' report of their awareness of their child's experience of PTSD symptoms. Significant differences were found between the child's self-report and the parents' report of PTSD symptoms, including intrusive thoughts, reliving/flashbacks, psychological distress at symbolic events, avoidance of activities, estrangement from others, and physiological distress at symbolic events. In each case, the surviving sibling's self report of the above-stated symptoms exceeded the parents' rating. Applebaum and Burns (1991) report that this occurrence may be caused by two factors: (1) parents' absorption with their own symptoms resulted in failure to notice the suffering of their children and (2) the children's reported desire to shelter their parents from any additional pain. Ultimately, it is reported that the PTSD symptoms experienced by both siblings and parents may result in a "contagious" spread of the PTSD symptoms from parent to child and from child to parent.

Rinear (1988) studied the psychosocial aspects of parental response patterns to the death of a child by homicide. This survey research found that "symptoms characteristic of PTSD began within 1 week of the child's murder and persisted for as long as 1 to 2 years thereafter" (p. 309). Masters, Friedman, and Getzel (1988) report that their clinical observations support "Rinear's findings that the families experienced most of the symptoms of post-traumatic stress syndrome: sleeplessness, nightmares, fatigue, startle reactions, phobias and fears involving situations associated with the murder" (p. 114). These findings supported Rinear's original hypothesis that the symptoms/reactions of the parents of murdered children would "fail to conform fully to any currently existent models of grief and mourning, but rather, would reveal characteristics of Post-Traumatic Stress Disorder" (p. 308).

Barnes (1995) polled experts (i.e., ICU nurses, physicians, social workers, psychologists, family therapists) who work with physically traumatized children on pediatric intensive care units (PICUs) to determine their views concerning family response patterns associated with the traumatic event and the ICU hospital experience. Findings indicate that experts identify family response patterns that demonstrate symptoms of a secondary traumatic stress reaction throughout the post-trauma and ICU experience.

These findings support Figley's (1995) contentions that the symptoms exhibited would be similar to the primary victim's, but with a focus on the primary victim rather than the specific traumatic event. The experts described family response patterns that were consistent with each DSM-IV criterion (APA, 1994), but that were focused on the possibility that the child may die, anxiety associated with a prognosis of permanent disability, fears about the unknown, specific injuries, denial of the reality of the consequences of the event, etc.

Barnes (1995) also reports that the sources of stress identified by the experts, specific to the PICU, are primarily associated with family concerns about the child's injuries and family issues of safety, trust, and a sense of personal control. While the family member's focus on the child's injuries and medical needs appears to be the continuation of the discussion from the previous paragraph, the family issues of trust, safety, and control appear to be significant trauma-related responses.

In support of the significance of the issues of trust, safety, and control for family members of physically traumatized children on the PICU, the collaborators identify several stressors. These stressors include family members' beliefs about personal and family vulnerability, attempts to convince other family members that everything is going to be alright, repeatedly asking the same questions over and over, concerns about having questions answered in a timely fashion, difficulty with frequent alarms going off in the child's room for no apparent reason, continued focus on all possible consequences of the child's injuries, the inability to develop trusting relationships with specific care-givers, and the tendency for family members to identify one specific care-giver who provides the type of care that they feel comfortable with and comparing all other care-givers to the standards set by that particular care-giver.

The collaborators also suggest that parents often experience a loss of control when they are required to turn over the care of their child to the ICU medical staff. Family members' preoccupation with the cause of the traumatic event and the child's medical condition may be attempts at regaining some sense of control in their lives.

Finally, Barnes (1995) proposes that family members' attempts to deal with multiple stressors associated with the traumatic event, life-threatening injuries, and the PICU experience result in a cumulative experience of systemic traumatic stress reaction within the family system. The collaborators in this study clearly supported the belief that family members demonstrate affective, cognitive, and behavioral changes following the traumatic event. They also supported the belief that the stable relationships between family members necessarily change in response to the individual changes mentioned above and the demands for the care of the injured child. The use of the term "systemic traumatic stress" appears to be most appropriate for the sudden demands that are being imposed on each member of the family system and the changes in interactional relationships that result (Barnes, 1995).

A REVIEW OF CHILD-BASED LITERATURE

As stated earlier in this chapter, there is minimal traumatology literature that addresses the relationship between childhood trauma and its influence on the victim's family system. In order to expand the knowledge base concerning parental secondary traumatization, the search was expanded to include literature from nursing, family medicine, and pediatric cancer.

Nursing

From the nursing literature, one research article was identified (Miles, 1985) that dealt with family response patterns following the death of a child. A significant finding from this study is that the amount of "perceived stress" and parental experience of lower socioeconomic status were the most influential factors on the degree of emotional sequelae experienced by the parent. When one considers the role that individual and family perceptions concerning the traumatic or stressful event play in the cognitive models of PTSD and in the family stress theories, it may be significant that the family's perceived stress after the death of a child would be more influential on symptom development than actual, observable life stressors.

A theoretical paper by Shaw and Halliday (1992) supports the proposition that family perception of crisis is a major influencing factor in how a family will respond to crisis. Ultimately, it is proposed that in chronic illness, the crisis is not the problem, but it is the family's "constraining beliefs that restrict alternative views about the crisis that becomes the problem" (Shaw & Halliday, 1992, p. 541). According to the authors, the family's response to the crisis event will be determined by the frame of reference through which they perceive the crisis. Figley (1988) agrees that perception plays a major role in the family response to a traumatic event and proposes that families that maintain or construct a more positive world view associated with the crisis or traumatic event will deal with it in a more positive manner.

Family Medicine

As in the nursing literature, family perception as a primary factor in family members' response to chronic illness in a child is strongly supported in each of the following articles identified in the family medicine literature. Gallo (1991) and Thompson, Gustafson, Hamlett, and Spock

(1992) both studied family response patterns to chronic, life-threatening pediatric illnesses and found that family perceptions play a large role in the family choice of coping mechanisms. Thompson et al. (1992) propose that psychological distress of the parents of chronically ill children is explained more by their perceptions and low inter-family support than by the actual medical condition of the child. Again, the family members' cognitive response to the circumstances surrounding the child's illness and the influence of these cognitive responses on family interactional patterns are found to be more influential on the family's experience of psychological distress than the child's actual physical condition.

Childhood Cancer

The diagnosis of childhood cancer clearly results in family system changes that are similar to those identified in the adult traumatology literature. Two research articles (Koch, 1985; Madan-Swain, Sexson, Brown & Ragab, 1993) from the literature pertaining to pediatric cancer were found that address family response patterns.

Koch (1985) identified five consistent themes in his qualitative study of the parents of pediatric cancer patients:

1. An increase in negative affect is associated with the family's concerns about the possible death of their sick family member and the impact that the illness will have on each family member's life.
2. Rules prohibiting emotional expression associated with the illness were quickly developed, supporting the family's repression or denial of the issues described in the first theme.
3. Frequent health and behavior problems developed in family members, other than the cancer patient, after the diagnosis of cancer (i.e., alcoholism, extramarital affairs, suicide attempts, hepatitis, death in automobile accidents, etc.).
4. Role changes occurred after the diagnosis of cancer. Often, the parents' primary focus was on the cancer patient. This resulted in siblings receiving less attention and acting out as a reaction to the role change. Often siblings were placed in adult caretaker roles, which resulted in rapid increases in reported sibling maturity. Another role change took place as siblings began to assume the role of emotional caretaker for their parents by hiding painful feelings and fears from parents.

5. Families reported the belief that the challenge of this family crisis had brought the family closer and had strengthened the family's cohesiveness.

The Madan-Swain et al. (1993) study investigated the coping and adaptation skills of siblings of childhood cancer patients. The findings of this study appear to support Koch's (1985) findings associated with role changes. Older siblings reportedly assumed parental roles and caretaker responsibilities, which seemed to blur the parent–child boundaries and result in the siblings' perception of being withdrawn from and less involved in family activities. Additionally, the bond that is established between the cancer patient and parents through the period of medical treatment serves to further isolate the other siblings from the parents and the cancer patient.

AXIOMS ASSOCIATED WITH THE SECONDARY TRAUMATIZATION OF PARENTS

It was stated earlier that a primary goal of this chapter is to identify testable axioms associated with the secondary traumatization of parents. Popper (1965) defines axioms as either conventions or scientific hypotheses. This chapter concludes with a discussion of the axioms that have been identified in the literature associated with family response patterns following the traumatization, death, or illness of a child family member. These axioms are the foundation upon which our understanding of this process of secondary traumatization and future research questions must be built.

1. Following the traumatization of a child, the parents and siblings will report having experienced emotional, cognitive, and behavioral symptoms that are similar to those reported by primary victims of PTSD. These trauma response patterns reported by the parents of traumatized children will be qualitatively different from existing models of grief. The PTSD symptoms that have been reported in the literature (Applebaum and Burns, 1991; Rinear, 1988) on parents of traumatized children include intrusive thoughts, nightmares, flashbacks, feeling of detachment or estrangement from others, restricted affect, emotional and physiological distress associated with the traumatic event, avoidance

of activities that remind the family of the child's traumatization, sleeplessness, startle reactions, and fatigue.

2. The focus of the parents' secondary trauma symptoms will be maintained on the experiences and physical or emotional condition of the primary trauma victim. Barnes (1995) speaks to this issue at length when he supports Figley's (1995) contention that secondary traumatic stress reactions will be focused on issues associated with the primary trauma victim's physical and emotional condition. Koch (1985) addresses this issue when he proposes that increased negative affect is associated with parental concerns about the child's critical condition and its effects on the siblings of the cancer patient. Koch (1985) and Madan-Swain et al. (1993) both discuss the preoccupation that parents maintain with the ill child, at the expense of their relationship with the other siblings.

3. Parental world view associated with personal vulnerability, safety, and control will be altered as a result of the child-traumatizing event. Barnes (1995), who found this to be a significant finding in his study, was the only one in the review of secondary traumatic stress in parents to identify this axiom. This issue becomes more informative when one considers Janoff-Bulman's (1992) contention that alterations in the world view of the traumatized individual can directly influence the victim's experience of depression, intrusive thoughts, breakdowns in interpersonal trust, anger, rage, feelings of vulnerability, disillusionment, lost sense of safety, and loss of self-worth and self-confidence.

4. Parental perceptions associated with the amount of stress resulting from the traumatizing event will influence their interactional patterns, selection of coping mechanisms, and the degree of emotional sequelae experienced by the parents. This point is strongly supported in the research by Gallo (1991), Miles (1985), and Thompson et al. (1992). Parental perceptions appear to play a major role in the recovery process for families as well. Koch (1985) proposes that many families believed that the challenge of the crisis resulted in a more cohesive and emotionally closer family, while Figley (1988) suggests that families that are able to recognize the strengths they have developed through their struggles following the traumatic event are better able to recover from their experience of secondary trauma.

5. The traumatization of a child family member will cause sufficient alterations in family organization that the family will experience major changes in the communication patterns and role behaviors. Applebaum and Burns (1991), Koch (1985), and Madan-Swain et al. (1993) all agree that parents and siblings of the traumatized child experience role changes that serve to protect the parents, while alienating the siblings from the parents and the primary trauma victim. Older siblings often assume the role of adult caretaker of younger children in order to free the parents up to care for the primary trauma victim. A second role change again includes the older siblings, who assume the role of emotional caretaker for their parents.

6. Multiple stressors resulting from the immediate needs of the parents, siblings, and traumatized child will result in a systemic traumatic stress reaction among family members. Barnes (1995) reports that a traumatizing event may result in immediate stressors that can impact the lives of all family members for days, weeks, months, or years. This wound to the family system may impact much more than the family's life routines and may be observable through disruptions in the family members' stable patterns associated with behavior, communication, discipline, and emotional support. The expert collaborators in the Barnes (1995) study agreed that failure on the part of the family to deal with these disruptions in family interactional patterns will ultimately result in arguments, resentments, and attention-getting behaviors between family members. If the systemic stressors continue to go unattended, noticeable patterns of triangulation and blaming become common family dynamics.

CONCLUSION

If there is accuracy in the axioms that were identified in the literature associated with the families of traumatized or critically ill children, then it may be appropriate to assume that many of the family members of traumatized children experience a significant disturbance in individual and systemic functioning, which begins almost immediately following the traumatizing event. These findings appear significant in that they indicate the need for the availability of immediate and carefully conceptualized interventions for these family members in need, as early as possible in the post-trauma phase of their child's treatment. It may be hypothesized that those families that do not receive the needed therapeutic assistance will continue to experience difficulty throughout the years to come. Many of these families may make their way into family therapy for the system difficulties that are directly related to the systemic traumatic stress response. Other family members may make their way into individual psychotherapy to deal with their own secondary traumatic stress response. It is important for the therapist at both therapeutic junctions to be aware of the relationship between the secondary and systemic traumatization that results from the parents' experiences associated with the traumatization of a child.

In Chapter 7 in this book, Barnes (1996) draws on the axioms identified in this chapter to discuss effective treatment methods for families suffering from secondary traumatization. Structural, cognitive, and developmental models of family therapy are discussed as useful models for assisting families in dealing with changes in cognitive beliefs about the family and the traumatizing event, as well as systemic alterations in family structure.

REFERENCES

American Psychiatric Association. (1994). *Diagnostic and Statistical Manual of Mental Disorders* (4th ed.). Washington, DC: American Psychiatric Association.

Amick-McMullan, A., Kilpatrick, D.G., Veronen, L.J., & Smith, S. (1989). Family survivors of homicide victims: Theoretical perspectives and an exploratory study. *Journal of Traumatic Stress, 2*(1), 21–35.

Applebaum, D.R., & Burns, G.L. (1991). Unexpected childhood death: Posttraumatic stress disorder in surviving siblings and parents. *Journal of Clinical Child Psychology, 10*(2), 114–120.

Barnes, M.F. (1995). *The Impact of the Physical Traumatization and Critical Care Hospitalization of Children, on the Functioning of the Injured Child's Family System: A Delphi Study*. Unpublished doctoral dissertation. Tallahassee: Florida State University.

Barnes, M.F. (1997). Treating burnout in families following childhood trauma. In C.R. Figley (Ed.), *Burnout in Families: the Systemic Cost of Caring* (pp. 169–183). Delray Beach, FL: St. Lucie Press.

Burr, W.R., Klein, S.R., & Associates (1994). *Reexamining Family Stress: New Theory and Research*. Thousand Oaks: Sage Publications.

Carroll, E.M., Rueger, D.R., Foy, D.W., & Donahoe, C.P. (1985). Vietnam combat veterans with posttraumatic stress disorder: Analysis of marital and cohabitating adjustment. *Journal of Abnormal Psychology, 94*(3), 329–337.

Feinauer, L. (1982). Rape: A family crisis. *The American Journal of Family Therapy*, *10*(4), 35–39.

Figley, C.R. (1983). Catastrophe: An overview of family reactions. In C.R. Figley and H.I. McCubbin (Eds.), *Stress and the family, Volume II: Coping with catastrophe* (pp. 3–20). New York: Brunner/Mazel.

Figley, C.R. (1986). Traumatic stress: The role of the family and social support system. In C.R. Figley (Ed.), *Trauma and its wake, Volume II: Traumatic stress theory, research and intervention* (pp. 39–54). New York: Brunner/Mazel.

Figley, C.R. (1988). Treating traumatic stress in family therapy. *Journal of Traumatic Stress*, *1*, 1.

Figley, C.R. (1989). *Helping traumatized families*. San Francisco: Jossey-Bass.

Figley, C.R. (1990). Post-traumatic family therapy. In F.M. Ockberg (Ed.), *Post-traumatic therapy and victims of violence* (pp. 83–109). New York: Brunner/ Mazel.

Figley, C.R. (1992). Secondary traumatic stress and disorder: Theory, research and treatment. Paper presented at the First World Meeting of the International Society for Traumatic Stress Studies, Amsterdam.

Figley, C.R. (1993). Compassion stress: Towards its measurement and management. *Family Therapy News,* January, 3,16.

Figley, C.R. (1995). Compassion fatigue as secondary traumatic stress disorder: An overview. In C.R. Figley (Ed.), *Compassion fatigue: Secondary traumatic stress disorder in treating the traumatized.* New York: Brunner/Mazel.

Gallo, A.M. (1991). Family adaptation in childhood chronic illness: a case report. *Journal of Pediatric Health Care*, *5*(2), 78–85.

Hill, R. (1949). *Families under stress.* New York: Harper.

Janoff-Bulman, R. (1985). The aftermath of victimization: Rebuilding shattered assumptions. In C.R. Figley (Ed.), *Trauma and its wake: The study and treatment of post-traumatic stress disorder* (pp. 15–35). New York: Brunner/Mazel.

Janoff-Bulman, R. (1992). *Shattered assumptions: Towards a new psychology of trauma.* New York: The Free Press.

Jones, R.W., & Peterson, L.W. (1993). Post-traumatic stress disorder in a child following an automobile accident. *The Journal of Family Practice*, *36*(2), 223– 225.

Kisher, G.R. (1984). *Chiasmal effects of traumatic stressors: The emotional cost of support.* Unpublished thesis. West Lafayette, IN: Purdue University.

Koch, A. (1985). "If only it could be me": The families of pediatric cancer patients. *Family Relations*, *34*, 63–70.

Kulka, R.A., Schlenger, W.E., Fairbanks, J.A., Hough, R.L., Jordan, B.K., Marmar, C.R., & Weiss, D.S. (1990). *Trauma and the Vietnam War generation: Report of findings from the national Vietnam veterans readjustment study.* New York: Brunner/Mazel.

Lipovsky, J.A. (1991). Posttraumatic stress disorder in children. *Family Community Health*, *14*(3), 42–51.

Madan-Swain, A., Sexson, S.B., Brown, R.T., & Ragab, A. (1993). Family adaptation and coping among siblings of cancer patients, their brothers and sisters, and nonclinical controls. *The American Journal of Family Therapy*, *21*(1), 60–70.

Masters, R., Friedman, L.N., & Getzel, G. (1988). Helping families of homicide victims: A multidimensional approach. *Journal of Traumatic Stress 1*(1), 109–125.

McCann, I.L., & Pearlman, L.A. (1990). Vicarious traumatization: A framework for understanding the psychological effects of working with victims. *Journal of Traumatic Stress, 3*(1), 131–149.

McCubbin, M.A. & McCubbin, H.I. (1989). Theoretical orientations to family stress and coping. In C.F. Figley (Ed.), *Treating stress in families* (pp. 3–34). New York: Brunner/Mazel.

McCubbin, M.A. & Patterson, J.M. (1983). Family transitions: Adaptation to stress. In H.I. McCubbin & C.F. Figley (Eds.), *Stress and the family, Volume I.: Coping with normative transitions* (pp. 5–25). New York: Brunner/Mazel.

Miles, M.S. (1985). Emotional symptoms and physical health in bereaved parents. *Nursing Research, 34*(2), 76–81.

Mio, J.S., & Foster, J.D. (1991). The effects of rape upon victims and families: Implications for a comprehensive family therapy. *The American Journal of Family Therapy, 19*(2), 147–159.

Popper, K.R. (1965). *The logic of scientific discovery.* New York: Harper & Row.

Rinear, E.E. (1988). Psychosocial aspects of parental response patterns to the death of a child by homicide. *Journal of Traumatic Stress, 1*(3), 305–322.

Rosenheck, R. (1986). Impact of posttraumatic stress disorder of World War II on the next generation. *The Journal of Nervous and Mental Disease, 174*(6), 319–327.

Rosenheck, R., & Nathan, P. (1985). Secondary traumatization in the children of Vietnam veterans with post-traumatic stress disorder. *Hospital Community Psychiatry, 36*, 538–539.

Semonin-Holleran, R. (1991). Pediatric trauma patients: Differences and implications for emergency nurses. *Journal of Emergency Nurses, 17*(1), 24–31.

Shaw, M.C., & Halliday, P.H. (1992). The family, crisis and chronic illness: An evolutionary model. *Journal of Advanced Nursing, 17*, 537–543.

Silver, S.M., & Iacono, C. (1986). Symptom groups and family patterns of Vietnam veterans with post-traumatic stress disorder. In C.R. Figley (Ed.), *Trauma and its wake, Volume II: Traumatic stress theory, research and intervention* (pp. 78–96). New York: Brunner/Mazel.

Solomon, Z., Mikulincer, M., Freid, B., & Wosner, Y. (1987). Family characteristics and posttraumatic stress disorder: A follow-up of Israeli combat stress reaction casualties. *Family Process, 26*(3), 383–394.

Solomon, Z., Waysman, M., Levy, G., Freid, B., Mikulincer, M., Benbenishty, R., Florian, V., & Bleich, A. (1992). From front line to home front: A study of secondary traumatization. *Family Process, 31*, 289–302.

Thompson, R.J., Gustafson, K.E., Hamlett, K.W., & Spock, A. (1992). Stress, coping, and family functioning in the psychological adjustment of mothers of children and adolescents with cystic fibrosis. *Journal of Pediatric Psychology, 17*(5), 573–585.

TREATING STSD
IN CHILDREN

5

Mary Beth Williams, Ph.D.

INTRODUCTION

Children have what Terr (1990) termed "close encounters" with trauma in their everyday lives. Traumatic encounters range from rather small, indirect exposures (through the media, self-report of others) to direct exposures to the post-traumatic symptoms of others (particularly if those others are friends, parents, or close acquaintances) to exposure to post-traumatic symptoms in others. Close encounters may change the lives of those exposed (Bell, 1991) and, as Samaroff, Siefer, Barocas, Zax, and Greenspan (1987) stated, few escape risk of exposure. Terr (1990) also added that a child does not have to be in the vicinity of the event to be traumatized by that event and needs only to imagine what it would be like to encounter the trauma and its aftereffects.

The short-term and long-term effects of trauma, therefore, are not confined to those who experience the events directly. Persons who care for, work with, know, are involved with, listen to the stories of, or even observe as bystanders or media viewers traumatized individuals may also experience symptoms of trauma, known as secondary symptoms. These secondary symptoms, when they conform to the DSM-III-R definition (1987), may constitute a secondary stress reaction with commonly recognized components of intrusion, avoidance/numbing, and increased physiological arousal. Secondary exposure to a traumatic event may undermine basic safety and trust in a just world (Erikson, 1963, 1967;

1-57444-047-0/98/$0.00+$.50
© 1998 by CRC Press LLC

Janoff-Bulman, 1992; McCann & Pearlman, 1990). Therefore, children who are exposed to the traumas of others may begin to question their own personal safety and may be therefore less trusting of the world and those in that world. The extent of the secondary reaction depends upon a number of factors. The type of trauma, number of traumas, extent and degree of indirect exposure or direct exposure to the symptoms of others, the length of exposure, whether or not exposure is repetitive (and, hence, cumulative), age at the time of exposure, and the developmental stage of the child are several. Additional factors include the coping abilities, capacity for resilience, problem-solving abilities, beliefs about the event and its meaning, locus of control, help-seeking strategies (including involvement in proactive organizations such as SADD), and the number and involvement of social support systems. Figure 5.1 presents these factors in diagrammatic format. As Terr (1990) noted, however, it is the context of the traumatic event which often makes the major difference. Rutter (1987) found that secondary traumatic reactions are more likely to occur if multiple risks for exposure are present.

This chapter examines a number of events which can lead to secondary traumatic stress reactions when children are exposed to them. A primary emphasis is the exposure of children to the post-traumatic symptoms of their family members in general and parents in particular. Parental symptoms may be the result of domestic violence; exposure to war and combat; incarceration during war; or a history of early physical, sexual, or emotional abuse. This chapter considers the developmental implications of secondary post-traumatic stress reactions; suggests ways to assess the level of impairment of children who are secondarily traumatized; and proposes school-related, individual, and family-oriented treatment methods.

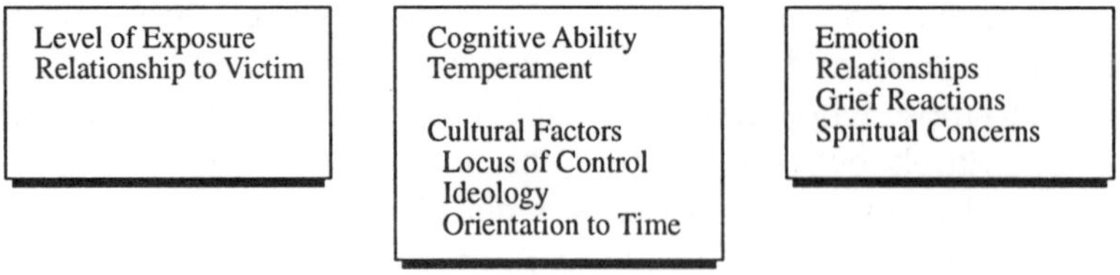

Level of Exposure Relationship to Victim	Cognitive Ability Temperament
	
	Cultural Factors
	  Locus of Control
	  Ideology
	  Orientation to Time
		Emotion Relationships Grief Reactions Spiritual Concerns

Figure 5.1   Factors in Diagrammatic Format

TRAUMATIC EVENTS THAT LEAD TO SECONDARY REACTIONS

Serious Illness Leading to Death; Death by Suicide or Homicide

Friends and classmates of children whose parents are incapacitated by a life-threatening illness, have died, or have been killed are suddenly thrust, depending on their developmental level, into an awareness that life is not permanent. If death or terminal illness happened to the family member of a friend, it could also happen to one's own family member. Worden (1991) noted that children do mourn and, therefore, have the capacity to mourn for others who are mourning.

If the death was by suicide, it is possible that even more intense secondary reactions may occur. Johnson and Maile (1987) wrote that knowledge of a suicide leads children who are upper-elementary age and beyond to recognize the vulnerability of life. While primary survivors (those closest to the dead individual) often exhibit post-traumatic reactions, secondary reactions can extend to an entire student body, thereby changing the entire atmosphere of a school. Persons who are closely identified with these primary survivors (best friends, relatives) may experience more intense secondary reactions and may be more likely to question their own mortality. Their belief in invulnerability of the self turns to doubt (Steele, 1992). Even children who have only heard about the suicide fantasize about what it was like to die and keep scenes of that death in their minds for extended periods of time.

Homicide is becoming more frequent within the family. Over one-third of all murders are committed by one family member against another (Domestic Abuse, 1989). Survivors of murdered individuals frequently experience symptoms of secondary post-traumatic stress. These survivors have not necessarily witnessed the death. Secondary symptoms in these survivors may be even more intense than symptoms in survivors of persons who have died of natural causes because of the sudden, violent nature of homicide.

War

One of the first researchers to record secondary trauma among children exposed to war was Fields (1989) as she gathered data from "Children of the Intifada." According to Garbarino, Kostelny, and Dubrow (1991), children who live through or are exposed to war may be "missocialized into a model of fear, violence and hatred" because "war maims children, injures children," and teaches children that attachments can be disrupted. When children hear stories of war or see pictures of war, they are constantly reminded that other children have lost their parents, their homes, and even their countries. The Project on Children and the War, researching exposure of children to different levels of war, found that different exposure leads to different reactions (DeAngelis, 1992). The more children were directly or indirectly exposed to war-related events, the more likely they were to develop post-traumatic stress disorder (PTSD).

Children are also secondarily traumatized if their parents have been exposed to or have been participants in war. Rosenheck and Nathan (1985), studying secondary trauma in children of Vietnam veterans, found that children exposed to reliving experiences in their parents tend to identify with those parents and experience similar events in fantasy, internalizing a fearful reality. Children of veterans with PTSD tend to act out family pathology through emotional distancing, depression, and behavioral and school-related problems (Williams & Williams, 1987).

Sipprelle (1992) found that many trauma symptoms exhibited by Vietnam veterans are interpersonal in nature. For example, PTSD-positive veterans who demonstrate typical avoidant symptoms of constriction of interest, feeling of detachment, restricted affect, and irritability may impact their children by forcing them to either carry out activities without them (e.g., participation in sports or school activities) or remain in the home, experiencing secondary isolation. The PTSD-positive veterans' physiological reactions of hypervigilance and an exaggerated sense of danger may shape their children's beliefs about vulnerability and safety. In addition, the Vietnam veteran survivor often sees his/her role as that of protector and provider rather than lover or loving parent. Thus, choices of ways to express love, which may avoid true intimacy, often do not meet the needs for connection of children and may force children and partners to look elsewhere for expressions of affection or love (Sipperelle, 1992). Rosenheck and Nathan (1985) and Rosenheck (1986) noted that children of veterans who were emotionally close to their fathers appeared to absorb and carry paternal pain into their adult lives, impacting choice of partner, career, and lifestyle.

Sommer (1992) noted that not knowing the status of loved ones may lead to chronic uncertainty and secondary traumatic reactions for many families of POWs/MIAs, as these individuals fantasize about the fate of their loved ones. Lack of government cooperation and an unwillingness to release information have contributed to the secondary traumatic reactions of children of these POWs/MIAs and have led them to "do things on their own (e.g., going to Vietnam to investigate their fathers' or brothers' cases"). Angry, frustrated family members have testified before congressional committees, written articles, and appeared on television shows. Some have quit jobs and school to spend time attempting to resolve the fate of parents or siblings; others have committed suicide. Various support groups, including the National Alliance of Families, have been founded around the issue (Sommer, 1992).

In Touch is an organization founded in 1989 to help sons and daughters of deceased Vietnam veterans find one another and contact living veterans who knew their parents. Reconnections have helped to solve family mysteries and have assisted children, who are now adults, to complete their grieving process (Sommer, 1992). Participation in a recent five-hour open group discussion of Sons and Daughters in Arlington, Virginia by this author reinforced her recognition of secondary traumatic stress symptoms in these young adults. Many of the children of deceased veterans who were present discussed their attempts to find out "what their dads were like, how they died" and described what it was like to grow up in a house in which their remaining parent (mother) may have experienced secondary post-traumatic stress.

Neighborhood and Family Violence

Children learn to be violent by participating in or observing violence within their families (Straus, Gelles & Steinmetz, 1980, 1981) or their neighborhoods. Children can be impacted by observing violence of one parent toward another. In fact, children who have observed violence between parents are more likely to be violent in their own later marriages. Sixteen percent of all marriages have some form of physical violence within a given year, and 28% of women in marriage are hit over the course of those marriages.

Children's reactions to family violence have been targeted only recently. There have been no epidemiological studies of the incidence or prevalence of secondary trauma in children of battered women. Marital violence is a multithreat stressor which puts the victim at risk for injury and even death. Children involved in a violent family may feel helplessness, fear of (yet may also seek) family dissolution, and, according to Pynoos and Eth (1986a), are in a constant state of anxious arousal. These authors liken the violent family to a war zone. In fact, the greater the likelihood of the occurrence of marital rape, parental suicide, or parental murder, the greater the impact on those children. When children have witnessed the death of a parent from family violence, their grief and post-traumatic stress are even more severe (Wilson, Smith & Johnson, 1985).

Strauss, Gelles, and Steinmetz (1980) also noted, according to Barnett, Pittman, Ragan, and Salus (1980), that many children believe that they are the cause of the violence, even when they were not involved. Children who are secondarily exposed to violence, according to Richter (1991), lose a belief in a just, benevolent world. They place less value on human life, believe they are less likely to survive into adulthood, are less willing to develop and maintain relationships, and are less likely to commit prosocially. In addition, they often retreat into silence (Black & Kaplan, 1988).

Children are also increasingly being exposed to violence in their neighborhoods. Garbarino et al. (1991) reported that 14 of 19 13-year-old students in a Washington, D.C. classroom knew someone who had been killed by shooting, stabbing, or drugs. Every child in a sample of children living in public housing in Chicago had a firsthand encounter with shooting by age five (Dubrow & Garbarino, 1989). These children, as well as the acquaintances and friends who hear their stories, learn that they, too, have little control over the danger of their immediate environments. McNully (1994) concluded that exposure to violence was more likely to produce post-traumatic symptoms than were other types of traumatic events. As Pynoos and Nader (1988) noted, communities (and the children living in those communities) are "disturbed in a unique fashion by the occurrence of unexpected violence," and may experience secondary reactions which include fears of reoccurrence and ongoing "concerns about security, anger, and preoccupations with revenge."

Disasters

Green, Korol, Grace, Vary, Leonard, Gleser, and Smitson-Cohen (1991) noted that most studies of children who are exposed directly or indirectly to disasters have not focused on the presence or absence of PTSD. However, these researchers did recognize that children exposed to disasters were at risk for developing symptoms of PTSD. Parental functioning, they found, influenced the impact of the disaster. Children whose parents were less functional were more at risk for a post-traumatic reaction.

Children who are secondarily traumatized by disasters seek to process what they have seen, heard, or been told by others. If they, too, live in dysfunctional homes, their reactions may be more profound because supportive functions of caretakers may be limited. Catherall (1992) supported this finding by noting that if parents cannot support their children or are not stable, the children are more likely to develop secondary traumatic reactions.

Living with Parents Who Are Adult Survivors of Severe Childhood Trauma

Many adult survivors of severe childhood trauma (e.g., child abuse in general and sexual abuse in particular) suffer from symptoms of PTSD years after their abuse (Williams, 1990). The children and spouses of those survivors may be exposed to their symptoms and may suffer from secondary traumatic stress. Countless other children live in homes in which parents are survivors of physical child abuse, child neglect, or were witnesses to family violence. Catherall (1992) wrote that the effects of parental traumatization (whether as children or adults) are passed on to the children.

The families of these adult survivors are often dysfunctional. Parents may tend to close down in crises or perceive events to be crises when they are not, thereby contributing to the secondary traumas experienced by their children. They may not have appropriate empathy with the pain their children feel when either directly or indirectly traumatized. In many instances, these adults have not dealt with their own losses, lack energy to deal with others, and may have never disclosed their past traumatic experiences to their families.

When parental exposure to current traumatic events (or the impact of past traumatic events) impairs parental functioning in any way, it threatens family system functioning, may interfere with a variety of family activities in the arenas of work and play, and impacts children's stability and security. As Figley (1989) noted, the greater the adult's distress, the greater the distress in other family members. The distress becomes even more magnified if the primary victim of the traumatic event (in most cases the parent) further victimizes other family members through abuse and/or violence (e.g., physically, emotionally, or even sexually abusing children).

Children of parents with a history of trauma, particularly trauma that is severe in nature (e.g., exposure to atrocities, repeated sexual abuse, torture), exhibit a variety of secondary symptoms that may recapitulate the PTSD of the parent. They may exhibit symptoms of intrusion, avoidance, and physiological hyperarousal or hypervigilance. Specific secondary responses are described in the section examining developmental factors.

Rosenthal, Sadler, and Edwards (1987) noted that families in which parents are trauma survivors may exhibit the following symptom patterns:

1. Boundary distortions centering on individuation, intimacy, separation; children may be forced out of the nest early or not be allowed to separate
2. Somatization of the trauma experiences with their behavioral, emotional, cognitive, and sensory aspects (i.e., children may develop physical symptoms mimicking the parental trauma)
3. Role reversals wherein the children take on the roles of parents
4. Alienation toward the victim (once knowledge of victimization is gained)
5. Ambivalence toward the victim, not knowing if one loves or hates one's parent
6. Extreme need for social support sought in unhealthy ways, often from inappropriate peer or adult figures
7. Feelings of guilt, shame, self-blame
8. Self-destructive behaviors, including temper tantrums
9. Inappropriate attempts to control the survivor and the family through acting out, deflecting anger onto self as a means of control
10. Abusive language and behavior
11. Interruption of the normal developmental life cycle, causing regression, stagnation, or pseudo-adulthood
12. Overreactions to daily stressors

Albeck (1994) called these effects the "generational consequences of trauma." He noted, as well, that there is "still a great deal to learn about the influences parental traumas exert on the lives of their children during and after their formative years." Figley (1988) termed these secondary symptoms the "chiasmal effects" of trauma—reactions that impact and infect other family members.

Exposure to Traumatic Events Through the Media

Children are indirectly exposed to a variety of violent or otherwise traumatic events through television, movies, videos, newspapers, and magazines. Hurricane Andrew, which devastated southern Florida in late summer 1992, not only traumatized children in its path but children thousands of miles removed. As the aftermath of the hurricane swept through Virginia days later, children as old as 12 were afraid to be home alone and hid in the basement to protect themselves should the hurricane come there as well. No amount of reassurance could convince them that their homes were safe.

As Terr (1990) reported, the explosion of the *Challenger* space shuttle left psychological marks on children throughout the United States. The most common aftereffect was a fear of airplanes.

Although this description of potential traumatic events to which children are secondarily exposed is not complete, it does illustrate the fact that it is almost impossible to avoid some level of exposure. Secondary traumatic reactions are more intense, however, if the exposure is recurrent rather than a one-time event. A child who watched the *Challenger* disaster and then witnessed television coverage of an airplane crash, or learned that a relative of a friend died in an airplane crash, is much more likely to have secondary traumatic stress than is a child who watched the *Challenger* disaster only once. An eight-year-old child who lives in a family in which the mother has frequent flashbacks of childhood abuse is generally more likely to experience intense secondary stress symptoms than is a child whose parent was mugged on a street corner but was not injured. In addition, a solitary secondary exposure is generally more intense than is exposure that is shared and discussed.

The level of life threat experienced by primary survivors impacts their reactions and hence the reactions of those secondarily exposed—the greater the life threat and accompanying levels of pain, the greater the chance of secondary trauma (Webb, 1992). The impact of secondary exposure is also greater if that impact challenges or questions the child's self-esteem, ability to maintain positive and intimate relationships, internal locus of control, and dreams of the future. Steele (1992) noted that children do not become desensitized with repeated secondary exposures. They may appear to be indifferent or untouched but, internally, feel hopeless and helpless. Children who are secondarily exposed to a one-time trauma (what Terr [1991] termed Type I trauma) tend to process their reactions much more easily than do children who are repeatedly secondarily exposed to recurrent traumas (Type II traumas), particularly if those traumas are in their families.

DEVELOPMENTAL FACTORS

What individual characteristics of children influence whether or not the child develops a secondary reaction and the degree of that reaction? Shirk (1988) noted that age, cognitive ability, level of ego development, conceptualization of death, developmental stage, and other similar factors influence the experience of violence, the reaction to traumatic reactions of parents and others, coping responses, and the understanding of events. Selman (1980) similarly noted that a child's understanding of conflict is developmentally based.

The following sections of this chapter explore four general stages of child development: preschool (0–5), elementary (6–10), preteen (11–12), and adolescence (12–18). A general description of developmental tasks, based primarily on the works of Erikson (1963; 1967), is followed by the stage-specific conceptualization of death. A short summary of typical stage-related secondary traumatic symptoms concludes the description. The objective of this section is not to construct a new theory of child development but to summarize the effects of trauma on children of certain age groups, utilizing the psychosocial theory of development to indicate how exposure to secondary stress impacts ego identity and may lead to regressive behavior, may intensify the existing psychosocial crisis, or may lead to psychosocial acceleration and pseudo-maturation.

Preschool Children

Description

Preschool children are generally interested in the immediate rewards of behavior, and their understanding of conflict depends upon what they perceive to be its immediate consequences. Their major goal is to defend their own possessions or rights when faced with conflict (Selman, 1980). The well-adjusted preschool child has successfully resolved developmental crises of trust vs. mistrust and autonomy vs. shame and doubt (Erikson, 1963, 1967). The preschool child therefore has reasonable trustfulness toward others and trustworthiness toward the self. The child feels secure in the permanence of a nurturing object (generally the mother), has learned a beginning level of body control, and is beginning to explore the world (Erikson, 1963, 1967). The preschool child also has learned to exhibit some self-control without a loss of self-esteem and exhibits pride in being autonomous. He or she also grants autonomy to others. However, if the child has been traumatized in such a way that trust and autonomy are challenged, the child's ability to work through and resolve this general stage of development is impaired. If a child does not have family stability, the child's ability to find direction and purpose may be limited and the child will not move on to work through the stage of initiative vs. guilt or begin to form relationships outside the family (Erikson, 1963, 1967).

Preschool children who have grown up in homes where parents have been traumatized may not receive consistent parenting and also may not have resolved these stages successfully. Secondary traumatic reactions may have developed as a result of the inconsistency and poor quality of parent–child interactions, Traumatized parents, particularly those who have not had treatment and continue to have active post-traumatic stress reactions or PTSD, may be unable to guide the child's quest for autonomy and may place excessive restrictions or punishments upon the child, thereby overprotecting that child and denying him or her the chance to develop self-control. If parents do not answer the preschool child's questions about traumas they have encountered or others have experienced, the child may develop feelings of guilt instead of initiative. Consistency is frequently the exception in homes of adult survivors of trauma. Imitating inconsistent behaviors and roles that are based on post-traumatic responses of numbing or repetition can also lead to secondary reactions (Ackerman, 1983).

Preschool children express feelings primarily through play that is often spontaneous and communicate needs through words. Their active imaginations lead them to create visual images of what they believe others experienced (NOVA, 1990). Their behaviors and reactions tend to mimic others; if those others are adults survivors of trauma who are actively experiencing PTSD, the secondary reactions of the children often are similar in form (Eth & Pynoos, 1985b).

Understanding of Death and Grief Reactions

Preschool children see death as temporary. They "play dead" and recognize television or film characters who have "died" in one show as "alive" in another. They have fantasies concerning death that may involve magical thinking. In other words, they believe they can make things happen by wishing them to happen, including death or regeneration. Hindman (1989) termed these children "unaware children," children who do not have understanding or awareness of the true meaning of the reactions of others to which they have been exposed. They tend to idealize the person who has been lost (Worden, 1991). Their "unaware" reactions are normal for their age and stage of development. They do recognize that death has some permanent ramifications but have little coping capacity to deal with death or the reactions of others who are traumatized by death. Exposure to other children who have experienced death threatens their security (Vondra, 1991). Death is a departure but not a finality. The dead, many preschoolers believe, are still able to eat, play, or sleep (Beckman, 1990).

Secondary Traumatic Symptoms

Green et al. (1991) discovered that secondarily traumatized preschool children exhibited specific behavioral disturbances, including both trauma-specific and more generalized fears, aggressive behaviors, regression in toilet training, and distractibility. Their findings supported earlier findings by Burke et al. (1982). These secondarily traumatized preschool children also may exhibit frozen watchfulness, sleep disorders, delayed or regressed motor development, and repetitive talk and play as they attempt to find meaning from the experiences and symptoms of those to whom they are exposed. Their post-traumatic play may be a form of obsessive repetition used to relieve anxiety through reenactments of what they imagine to be the primary trauma, since they were not directly exposed (James, 1994).

Preschool children are extremely vulnerable to stories or reports of traumas or exposure to traumatic symptoms in family members if those symptoms threaten the loss of the secure, safe world. Their reactions often show a proneness to negative affect as they unlearn previously learned skills and behaviors. They withdraw as their anxiety grows. Hindman (1989) stated that "developmental delays and limitations" may prevent children from exhibiting secondary symptoms.

Elementary School Age Children

Description

Elementary children ages 6–11 are working through the stage of development known as industry vs. inferiority (Erikson, 1967). Children now are able to look back, criticize themselves and their behaviors, and are able to express self-disgust. Language is well developed. Thought processes use problem-solving techniques, and the child has a better understanding of time and space, with some sense of both the past and the future. Elementary-age children still view families as primary to filling their needs but are beginning to develop strong peer relationships (NOVA, 1990). School and neighborhood have become important to them. They have some appreciation of the psychological effects of conflict and want good relationships with others (Selman, 1980). These children are learning how to get busy with objects and be busy with others. Older elementary-age students have begun to think abstractly and can begin with hypotheses. They also have begun to introspect and process information through deductive reasoning.

Understanding of Death and Grief Reactions

Elementary-age children, by the time they are approximately ten years of age, recognize that death exists and is irreversible. They have become aware of their own mortality and have fears of death (Lagorio, 1991). These children seek facts about death; if they are not given information, they can develop secondary traumatic reactions in which their imagination allows them to create scenarios, and they may exhibit intrusive thoughts, dreams, and/or nightmares (Beckman, 1990). They understand the changes loss brings to others and experience secondary symptoms of confusion, anger, fear, and sadness. Children may also mourn the losses of others deeply and, as they mourn, become less interested in play and increase distance from friends as part of their avoidance behaviors (Pynoos & Nader, 1988). These isolating behaviors contrast with the normal developmental tasks of this stage of development: being with peers, developing peer relationships, and functioning in a school community (Erikson, 1963, 1967).

Worden (1991) noted that, in order to understand death, children must comprehend the time concept of forever and concepts of irreversibility and transformation. Exposure to death threatens security, as these children take everything literally and try to make concrete connections between reactions and events. Giving children clear explanations of death at this age is essential. While children between the ages of six and nine tend to personify death as a "bad person" and may have a morbid interest in death, children by approximately age ten begin to view death as a universal, natural part of life.

Secondary Traumatic Symptoms

Terr (1991) noted that secondary symptoms develop when children realize that trauma to others may result in a loss of control of their own lives. Their sense of the future is affected, and they feel powerless to help those who are directly affected by the trauma. As noted earlier, children who witnessed the explosion of the *Challenger* space shuttle while at school experienced little behavioral reenactment of the event but had flashbulb memories of the disaster and replayed it through fantasy and visualizations (Terr, 1990b). Davidson and Smith (1990) reported that children who experience traumatic events prior to age 11 are three times more likely to develop PTSD than children who experience similar events after age 12.

Regressive secondary symptoms (symptoms by which children exhibit behaviors associated with an earlier psychosocial stage of development) continue to be common (e.g., excessive clinging and crying or engaging in previously extinguished habitual behaviors) (Erikson, 1967). Children who live in homes with traumatized parents may become irritable and aggressive. They may have specific fears or triggers which "set off" rage reactions or dissociative reactions in their parents. They may have elaborate nightmares, dreams, or fantasies about the events their parents experienced. Pynoos and Nader (1988) found, in their study of children exposed to community violence, that traumatic dreams were common ways to reexperience the violence secondarily.

The extent of direct reenactments present in those dreams depends on the degree of direct exposure to traumatic symptoms of others or traumatic events. Secondary reactions include more general fears of recurrence of violence than direct images of personal life threat. These common fears contribute to the secondary spread of traumatic symptoms; Terr (1985) called it "symptom contagion." Elementary-age children also experience feelings of survival guilt, particularly if "some specific action of theirs increased the threat to others" (Pynoos & Nader, 1988, p. 451).

School-age children may lose interest in school and may report or demonstrate problems of concentration. Pynoos and Nader (1988) did not observe children directly reporting that they felt numb. However, they did express feeling "more distant" from others or "more alone with their feelings" or "not wishing to be aware of their feelings."

Startle reactions, nervous reactions, and jumpiness are also typical. These children may appear to be hyperactive and frequently are diagnosed as attention deficit/hyperactive disorder (APA, 1987). They may have sleep problems, as they are anxious and hyperalert to family changes. These children may fantasize retributions toward those whom they perceive to be responsible for their parents' problems. Their psychosomatic complaints may be many, and their defenses may become more primitive as they split or dissociate themselves.

Ackerman (1983) wrote that children from alcoholic homes (or homes in which parents have been otherwise traumatized either as adults or children) attempt to alleviate the problems exhibited by their parents. However, when their efforts invariably fail, they begin to feel useless and are less likely to attempt to achieve in school. Impulse control may also become impaired, particularly if any sense of stability or routine is threatened. Thus, children who grow up in homes in which parents have been traumatized, or when secondarily exposed to traumas in others (through the media, friends, etc.), may display more serious secondary reactions than would be expected if they were from non-traumatized families. These reactions might include limit testing, obsessive play, secrecy about what "really goes on" in their lives, and poor self-concept. The avoidance component of those reactions might include withdrawal from peer and play groups. Secondary reactions are also evident while parents are in treatment but tend to decrease as parents heal, particularly if children are included in the treatment process via family and even individual sessions (Williams, 1992).

The Preadolescent and Adolescent

Description

The preadolescent has advanced language capabilities, but not necessarily advanced understanding of language concepts. He or she may tend to be judgmental about the world and self and may communicate by "acting out." The primary need of the preadolescent is support and self-esteem, and the primary center of relationships vacillates between family and peers (Erikson, 1963, 1967; NOVA, 1990). Preadolescents are entering the stage of Identity vs. Identity Diffusion as they attempt to integrate a social identity and consolidate a social role. According to Erikson's psychosocial theory of development, between the ages of 12–

20, young persons' major developmental tasks center around internalizing moral judgment, experimenting with roles of work and play, developing a sexual identity, learning to make decisions, and finding themselves primarily through interactions with others of their own age. This stage is often characterized by rapid physiological change as well as rapidly changing values and primary relationships.

Hindman (1989) noted that the most typical response of adolescents to trauma is one of outrage. Adolescents can use language creatively and communicate through a variety of modes and media, including drama, poetry, and art. They understand concepts of "cause and effect," tend to view events in terms of "black and white," and can explore possibilities without having to experience them directly. Adolescents are able to use symbolic thought and frequently fail to consider the consequences of their actions (NOVA, 1990; Erikson, 1963, 1967).

Understanding of Death and Grief Reactions

Preadolescents and adolescents understand the reality of death but may challenge its existence. They may defy death by taking risks as a means to control anxious fears. They also seek to find the meaning of life.

Secondary Traumatic Symptoms

According to Erikson's (1963, 1967) psychosocial theory of development, preadolescents often look to peers for reassurance and validation of their own perceptions and feelings. When secondarily traumatized, they may exhibit sleep and appetite disturbances as well as psychosomatic symptoms including headaches and breathing problems. They may question the fairness of what happened to others and are extremely self-judgmental. Some preteens express their guilt feelings over not being able to stop or control traumas that happen or happened to others through aggressive, rebellious behaviors, including sexual acting-out or substance abuse. Their secondary traumatic stress patterns of reactions begin to resemble those of adults.

Adolescents search for their own identities and meaning both individually and with the assistance of peer input and feedback. Their reactions are most similar to adult secondary reactions. They continue to be judgmental about their own and others' behaviors, including behaviors of their parents. They may even divert attention from themselves by triggering traumatic stress reactions in their parents. One 16-year-old, when her mother tried to implement rules and regulations in the home, lashed out verbally at her mother. The mother, upon hearing her daughter's tirades, generally reacted by having a flashback about her own abusive mother and was unable to follow through on the discipline. The mother became immobilized and the daughter proceeded to ignore the house rules. This situation and the accompanying triggers and transference components of the situation were addressed in an adjunct family therapy session. The mother was taught to recognize the daughter's manipulative pattern, and contracts concerning house rules were created.

Adolescents who grow up in a home replete with parental traumatic stress reactions may tend to be suspicious and guarded. They may be extremely self-conscious about their own vulnerability and do not want to appear to be "abnormal" to others. They may rarely invite friends to their homes and may even change peer groups or cease to associate with peers. Adolescents may use substances to numb themselves or may resort to self-mutilation or suicide thoughts, plans, and attempts to stop their pain. Teens who have been secondarily traumatized often have feelings of futurelessness, anxiety, apathy, and/or depression. Children whose parents have been abused as children often fantasize revenge toward the perpetrators and may assume a role of pseudo-maturity to compensate for parental immaturity (NOVA, 1990).

THE ROLE OF BELIEFS AND MEANING

The impact of secondary traumatic stress on children is mediated not only by the children's levels of resiliency and coping abilities, developmental stage, age, and level of exposure. It is also influenced by the perceived meaning of the traumatic event by the child. The roles of appraisal and belief systems concerning the impact of the trauma on safety, trust, power, esteem, and intimacy are central (McCann & Pearlman, 1990). Frequent secondary exposure to trauma can destroy the child's perception that the world is safe and trustworthy. The meaning of an event is very specific to a young child who views that event in a non-abstract way (Garbarino et al., 1992).

THE ROLES OF FAMILY AND ENVIRONMENTAL SUPPORT

The extent of a secondary traumatic stress reaction is also influenced by the reactions of parents to their traumatized children and the ability of those parents to provide support. Functional family systems have resources of cohesion, adaptability, trust, support, and mutual respect. Having a secure attachment to parents can help children cope more positively with later stress (Deangelis, 1992). Slaby (1989) identified seven stages of response that most families experience when dealing with a (secondarily) traumatized family member: uneasiness, reassurance-seeking, denial and minimizing, making the trauma survivor an outsider, feelings of guilt/shame/blame/grief, confusion over changes in the family, and acceptance of reality accompanied by a search for help. Even young children ages five or older are aware of these responses and may be involved with the healing process at any of these stages without commitment to helping.

The task of healing becomes even greater when more than one member of the family has experienced direct as well as secondary exposure to traumatic events. In many instances, children have parents who are veterans and/or have been sexually abused as children. One eight-year-old child who is exhibiting a severe secondary traumatic stress reaction has a stepfather who was a police officer shot in the line of duty. This man also is a survivor of physical abuse. The child's mother experienced sexual abuse by numerous perpetrators.

The abilities of these parents to provide support to their secondarily traumatized children may be limited, particularly if they have not had treatment themselves. Even during treatment for PTSD, their supportive roles may be limited, particularly if their focus tends to be primarily on their own healing (Williams, 1992). Matsakis (1989) noted that, in these marriages, parents tend to identify with each other and are so bound together through pain that their needs become foremost. In many of these families, the post-traumatic symptoms of parents have become the "norm" or have generalized to the children to become the expected manner of behavior for all family members. To a non-family member, these primary and secondary symptoms (nightmares, isolation, rage outbursts, sitting next to a wall, and scanning the setting) may seem weird or crazy. To the family members, they are normal.

McCubbin and Figley (1983) noted that the healthy family accepts the stressor as something that occurred outside the family setting and views symptoms as worthy of familial attention and assistance. Family members mobilize strengths and resources while exhibiting patience, tolerance, commitment, and affection. Communication among all family members is encouraged; the family "binds together" to offer support and assistance to the secondarily traumatized individual. Roles of all family members are more flexible to fit the demands of the situation at hand. Children seek information when needed, talk to external support systems when indicated, and openly process their own pain and distress. While emotional reactions are to be expected throughout the healing process, violent outbursts and/or substance abuse are not utilized as coping devices.

The role of the family must also be considered within the cultural framework of that family. What is the cultural belief about locus of control? What is the family's ideology, and how are stress and help-seeking viewed?

If parents do not provide stability and do not function as positive role models of coping and resilience, children need to have social support from extra-familial sources. It is important for all children to have positive relationships with adults within their communities, particularly if parents are impaired in their abilities to give support and encouragement. Teachers, counselors, school social workers, parents of friends, coaches, and others can be protective and provide positive support.

ASSESSMENT

A thorough assessment of children must be conducted prior to determining the type of treatment and the setting of treatment indicated for the secondarily traumatized child. If possible, it is important to ascertain the quality of non-trauma-related interactions of children with parents (Carroll, Foy, Cannon & Zweir, 1991) through either observation, self-report of the children, or individual conferences/meetings with the parents.

It is also important to assess through family and individual interviews the child's role or place in the family structure. The assessment seeks to determine how each child perceives his or her place in the family. The assessment examines the degree to which the child is responsible for caring for or doing the bidding of the parent or for protecting younger siblings, as well as what contributions each family member makes (Okun, 1984). The assessment examines the extent to which there are clear family boundaries concerning expression of affection, ventilation of anger or aggression, respect for individual privacy, and acceptance of responsibility. The degree to which children have been parentified, taking over the roles of the traumatized parent either by choice or by delegation, is also ascertained if possible.

There are a variety of paper-and-pencil assessment measures available to the clinician. Pynoos and Nader (1988) utilized a PTSD Reaction Index designed by Frederick (1985), as well as the Diagnostic Inventory for Children and Adolescents, to measure the extent of acute and chronic post-traumatic stress reactions in school-age children. James (1994) has designed a non-self-report instrument to measure the impact of sexual abuse trauma on children. Older children from age 12 onward, in the experience of this author, can complete the Trauma Symptom Checklist-33 (Briere & Runtz, 1987), the Impact of Events Scale (Horowitz, Wilbur & Alvarez, 1985), and the Williams-McPearl (TSI) Belief Scale (1991b). Another possible instrument is the 53-item Brief Symptom Inventory developed by Derogatis and Spenser (1982). Kulka et al. (1991) modified Achenbach's Childhood Behavior Checklist to develop a Childhood Behavior Problems Score. Gotbaum (1992) suggested using the Purdue PTSD Scale, a 15-item self-report measure that includes the 12 diagnostic PTSD criteria.

Families also vary in the amount and degree of disclosure of information that is permitted. When and how is it safe for children to tell others about their secondary reactions to trauma or their extent? Or, on the other hand, when is it safe for parents or other family members to reveal trauma histories to the children, and how is that telling to be done? If a family member has recently revealed to the parents that he or she is infected with the HIV virus, those parents must decide whether or not grandparents or siblings are to be told and what the risk of telling will be. If they are to be told, when and how is that information to be shared, and to what degree will their emotional reactivity be allowed, tolerated, or encouraged, valued, or devalued?

It is also important to assess how much secondary stress children can tolerate when their traumatized parent begins to work through what happened to him or her in flashbacks and/or abreactions. Therapists who work with survivors of trauma who are parents frequently do not consider the needs and reactions of the children of their clients. However, when a client recently attempted suicide after watching a nationally broadcast show for survivors of sexual abuse, this author included both husband and children in the session immediately following her release from the hospital. During that session, the secondary reactions of both husband and children were assessed and treatment was modified to include them. An adolescent who overheard her mother (who has a multiple personality disorder diagnosis) carry on a conversation with her father using a variety of voices expressed her symptoms of secondary trauma to her mother. The mother brought her to the subsequent session, where the extent of those symptoms were assessed. The child revealed that she had been having repeated fantasies and intrusive thoughts of her mother's earlier abuse based on the "bits and pieces" of conversations that she had heard. In this family, the child was encouraged to express her questions or emotions. Other families may not permit such open expression. If the family is not receptive to being involved in processing the secondary traumatic stress reaction, and if the child is not involved in individual treatment, then school staff may help the child, through a variety of groups, activities, and assignments, when programs are available.

Diagnosis and assessment of the child's secondary post-traumatic stress, for this author, is the funneling process that obtains information about the child's goals, presentation patterns, beliefs, coping abilities, levels of secondary exposure, and current symptom state. Short- and long-term treatment plans are based upon that diagnostic process as desired changes in behavior, emotional expression, belief systems, relationships, and somatic manifestations of the secondary impact are targeted.

McCann and Pearlman (1990) noted that it is important to assess the self-capacities and ego resources of all family members if family therapy is being considered. The following questions also need to be answered when the individual child is the client: How able is each child to tolerate strong affect in himself or herself and in others? To what extent does that child emotionally anesthetize himself or herself from the pain of the trauma? Is the child aware of his or her unmet needs that have been directly impacted by the trauma? How does the child get his or her needs met if those needs cannot be satisfied within the family system? To whom does the child turn for support, affection, attention, and intimacy? Can that child utilize or seek out alone time in order to rejuvenate, process what is occurring, or work on personal issues? In many instances, children who may exhibit secondary traumatic stress when alone are unable to handle isolation.

Is the child able to calm himself or herself when upset, frustrated, or feeling overwhelmed by constantly recurring crises? How does that child react if he or she falls short of personal expectations or the often constantly changing expectations of a traumatized parent? What are the beliefs of that child concerning safety, trust, power/independence, esteem, and intimacy (McCann & Pearlman, 1990)?

To what extent do family members blame themselves for the child's symptoms and reactions? Is this blame accurate or is it misdirected?

Does it involve self-loathing and potential suicidality, particularly if the parent is a trauma survivor? Suicide assessments must be conducted with all family members should any hint of self-destructive tendencies occur.

Adults who are trauma survivors frequently respond to family members, including their children, as if they were previous abusers. When this transference occurs, verbal and even physical attacks may coexist with episodes of externally directed rejection, rage, and anger or internally directed self-loathing. It is important to assess how children withstand angry outbursts and even physical outbursts (which are not to be tolerated). Another component of the assessment is to ascertain how much guilt and blame the children may assign to themselves or to the offending parent(s) for the situation, as well as the extent of compassion they have for that parent. Children should be asked where they find support and whether or not their parents encourage them to find support outside the home through school, sports, or activities. As Parson (1988) noted, it is important to evaluate whether or not family members are able to serve as part of the therapeutic support team for the traumatized child.

Murray and Kluckhorn (1953) identified a variety of ego resources for children and parents (even when the parents are trauma survivors themselves) that can help the child's healing process. These resources include intelligence, the ability to introspect, persistence, a fighting spirit, a strong sense of values, awareness of one's own psychological and emotional needs, the ability to distance self and gain perspective when necessary, and the ability to establish boundaries and make positive decisions. It is important to identify the presence or absence of these developmentally appropriate or inappropriate resources in each child who is participating in the therapeutic process (Erickson, 1963, 1967).

It is also extremely important to take a detailed trauma history of each child who participates in therapy (Pearlman & McCann, 1994). The existence of serious abuse, multiple victimizations, and exposure to violence and/or atrocity impacts the ability of a child to deal with the traumatic reactions of others, much less personal reactions. Figure 5.2 illustrates the diagnostic process.

TREATMENT

This section examines three specific areas of treatment: school-based interventions, individual treatment, and treatment for children who are

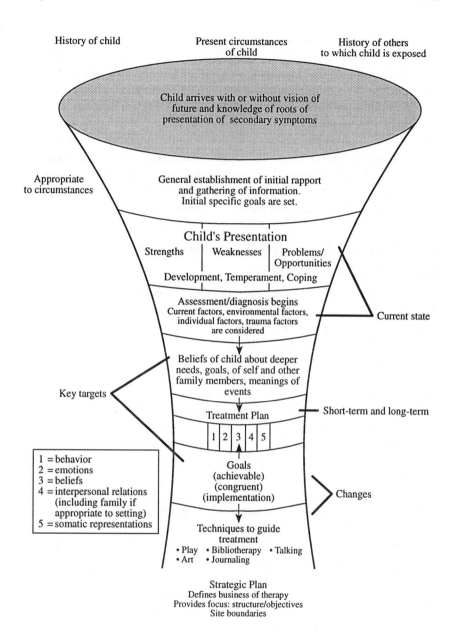

History of child   Present circumstances   History of others
                               of child   to which child is exposed

Child arrives with or without vision of
future and knowledge of roots of
presentation of secondary symptoms

Appropriate   General establishment of initial rapport
to circumstances   and gathering of information.
                         Initial specific goals are set.

Child's Presentation

Strengths | Weaknesses | Problems/
                         Opportunities

Development, Temperament, Coping

Assessment/diagnosis begins
Current factors, environmental factors,
individual factors, trauma factors
are considered
                                                    Current state

Beliefs of child about deeper
needs, goals, of self and other
family members, meanings of
events

Key targets

Treatment Plan   Short-term and long-term

1 | 2 | 3 | 4 | 5

1 = behavior   Goals
2 = emotions   (achievable)
3 = beliefs   (congruent)
4 = interpersonal relations   (implementation)   Changes
    (including family if
    appropriate to setting)
5 = somatic representations

Techniques to guide
treatment
• Play   • Bibliotherapy   • Talking
• Art   • Journaling

Strategic Plan
Defines business of therapy
Provides focus: structure/objectives
Site boundaries

Figure 5.2   The Diagnostic Process in Secondary Post-Truma Treatment

secondarily traumatized within their own families by parents who are trauma survivors.

In instances where diagnostic interviews reveal that children and/or a parent have poor ego resources and self capacities, where children are cognitively too young to be able to process the secondary trauma, or where there are ongoing episodes of violence or self-destructive behaviors or gestures within a family, family work is generally not appropriate. In these cases, it is more appropriate for the child to participate in individual or group therapy. If resources for individual treatment or group therapy are not available, however, the burden for intervention (though not for treatment) may fall upon the school.

School-Based Services to Alleviate Secondary Traumatic Stress Reactions

Garbarino et al. (1992) maintained that it is essential that the school take the role of a care-giving environment for traumatized children. Pynoos and Nader (1988), describing interventions with children who had been directly or indirectly exposed to community violence, stated that the school can be an ideal setting for classroom consultation and individual treatment."

Most schools, however, do not view themselves as therapeutic and prefer to restrict their interventions to counseling. Yet, sensitive schools can be a refuge for children, if they are predictable, organized, developmentally oriented, structured, and supportive (Garbarino, 1992). To be sure, this is not the primary purpose of the school—but it can be an indirect function of a well-designed program with caring teachers. A strategy for intervention in the school setting has been described by Williams (1994) elsewhere. A key aspect of intervention is to lessen the spread of trauma contagion by discussing what happened in the traumatic events that are of concern to the children (e.g., the violent death of a community leader or a teacher), while being extremely careful not to traumatize the children even further.

School-based activities can occur within the classroom or in smaller groups in the guidance counselor's office. A number of manuals have recently been created to address the needs of these students. Among them are *The Life Cycle Education Manual* (Lagorio, 1991); *Preventing Self Destruction: A Manual for School Crisis Response Teams* (Steele, 1992); *Suicide and the Schools: A Handbook for Prevention, Intervention and Rehabilitation* (Johnson & Maile, 1987); *Windows:*

Healing and Helping Through Loss (Hannaford & Popkin, 1992); and *Child Support (Through Small Group Counseling)* (Landy, 1988). The last book includes specific formats for children of divorce, children of incarcerated parents, and children of alcoholics, as well as death counseling, shyness counseling, and other topic areas. These manuals list a number of books by developmental stage that address issues of loss, death, violence, and grief. The books can be used by either the classroom teacher or other school professional (school social worker, psychologist, guidance counselor) with groups of students. Examples are *The Fall of Freddie the Leaf* (Buscaglia, 1982), *Charlotte's Web* (White, 1952), and *Nana Upstairs and Nana Downstairs* (DePaola, 1973).

Other classroom or school-based activities include the use of worksheets, writing assignments, or music and art assignments to address fears of contagion of secondary trauma; issues of death, grief, and loss; issues of worry about primary victims; and issues and/or traumas triggered by present events (Pynoos & Nader, 1988). Teachers and other school staff can also design structured or unstructured games to help children express feelings or resolve secondary traumatic stress reactions. Children may be assigned a journal and asked to write for a specific period of time either at home (if grade three or above) or in the classroom (kindergartners dictate to teachers, and first and second graders get assistance with words they cannot spell).

Guidance counselors, school social workers, or psychologists may lead ongoing groups for bereaved children or children of divorced parents, battered mothers, absent fathers, etc. These groups are generally topic-specific, help build skills, and are supportive rather than therapeutic in nature. Groups for children whose parents are trauma survivors can utilize material designed for partners of sexual abuse survivors as sources of topics or interventions (Gil, 1992; Landry, 1991; Davis, 1992; Hansen, 1992; Maltz & Holman, 1987; Graber, 1991; Spear, 1988; Dietz & Button, 1991a, 1991b; Williams, 1991a).

Groups have also been designed to help prevent secondary trauma in children whose mothers have been battered and who have fled (with those children) to shelters. Jaffe, Wilson, and Wolfe (1986a) used group interventions to help children understand and change attitudes toward family violence as well as develop strategies for conflict resolution. Alessi and Hearn (1984) designed group treatment for children in shelters. Malchiodi (1990) discussed the use of art therapy with children from violent homes. Roberts (1990) and Roberts and Roberts (1990) also described the use of coloring books for preschool and elementary-age children while they are in shelters. In fact, at the present time, most shelters have children's programs to help lessen the secondary traumatic impact (Ammerman & Hersen, 1990).

Individual Treatment for Secondary Traumatic Stress

Children need to be referred for treatment when they appear to be depressed or withdrawn, engage in self-destructive behaviors, have repeated psychosomatic (trauma-based) physical complaints, or act out excessively when other children who were similarly traumatized have moved on. Johnson (1989) noted that the signs that indicate the need for more intense intervention are generally cognitive (denial, out-of-control flashbacks, dissociation), emotional (uncontrolled crying, threats of harm to self or others, complete withdrawal), or behavioral (unfocused agitation, continual compulsive retelling of one's story, inability to care for oneself, destructive irritability).

Individual treatment for children may utilize play therapy involving puppets, art, dolls, stories, board games, and sand trays. Terr (1989) found that traumatized children tend to indulge in play at older ages than do non-traumatized children. According to Webb (1992), play therapy has six purposes. It aids diagnostic understanding, helps to establish the treatment relationship, is a medium for the child to work through defenses and handle anxiety, assists the child to verbalize feelings, helps the child act out unconscious material and relieve accompanying tensions, and enlarges the child's play interests. Play therapy alone may help to resolve secondary trauma in children who have had little exposure to limited traumas (Eth & Pynoos, 1985).

Teachers, as well as therapists, need to understand the meaning behind children's play, as well as its quality and "feel." Through play, children revise meanings, gain insight, and reduce anxiety. Play presents a means for children to try to make sense of the external reality of trauma in a symbolic way. Play is an empowering process.

Therapists can design age- and stage-specific interventions. For example, preschool and early elementary-age children, according to Pynoos and Nader (1988), need therapeutic intervention to help them verbalize general feelings, identify triggers, and to give them explanations about loss and death. The therapist helps to reestablish the protective shield around the child and assists in providing a caretaking function. In therapy, children are encouraged to reenact their traumatic reactions through play, puppet work, art, coloring books, bibliotherapy, singing, and reference to concrete props or visual aids. Repetition combined with physical activity helps relieve anxiety. Two series of workbooks for elementary- and secondary-age children by Alexander (1992, 1993) have been very helpful to this author. Each series of six workbooks deals with various types of trauma as well as both primary and secondary stress reactions. Examples of elementary-age books include *All My Feelings: A Story for Children Who Have Felt the Impact of Crime or Trauma, It Happened to Me: A Story for Child Victims of Crime or Trauma,* and *The World I See: A Story for Children Who Have Felt the Impact of Domestic Violence.* Books for teenagers include the following: *It Happened in Autumn: A Story for Teens Coping with a Loved One's Homicide, The Way I Feel: A Story for Teens Coping with Crime or Trauma,* and *When I Remember: A Story for Teens Who Have Witnessed Crime or Trauma.*

Early elementary-age children also utilize play with toys for reenactment and puppets to talk out their emotions, thoughts, and beliefs. Art therapy, bibliotherapy, story writing, behavioral rehearsals, journaling, and dream journaling assist in the resolution of secondary traumatic reactions. Children can be taught problem-solving skills as well as safety and prevention skills. Therapists can help these children express their imaginative fantasies about the events, identify triggers, act out reactions, report dreams, and develop methods of impulse control (Pynoos & Nader, 1988).

Preadolescents and adolescents need to be approached by therapists in a more adult manner. They can be taught about secondary traumatic stress responses and be helped to understand the various components of those responses. They are open to factual information and can also express their reactions in a proactive manner by becoming involved in community work or organizations. Therapeutic intervention can help lessen regression to earlier stages of development or acceleration into adulthood (Erikson, 1963, 1967). It is important for therapists to discuss any plans teens may have to avenge or revenge those who have been traumatized directly. Writing, journaling, poetry, artwork, and physical activity are all means to help resolve traumatic reactions. Kehayan (1990) noted that the goals of treatment for children grades 7–12 are to build self-awareness, self-esteem, social interaction, problem-solving and decision-making abilities, coping ability, ethical standards, creativity, and independent functioning.

Treatment for Children Whose Parents Are Trauma Survivors

Partners and children of trauma survivors may or may not be aware of the traumatic history of the parent, especially if that history has been repressed or dissociated. Sigal and Weinfeld (as found in Albeck, 1994) noted that children have various amounts of knowledge of the details of parents' lives. Sharing may have been inappropriate when it occurred or if it was prematurely or inadvertently delivered. (Albeck, 1994). Parents often do not reveal the extent of their traumatic experiences to their children. Children, therefore, may view the parent as being extremely volatile, unstable, unpredictable, hypervigilant, or avoidant without recognizing that those symptoms indicate a traumatic reaction. At some point, hopefully, the parent either reveals, faces (to some degree), or is forced by others to deal with the consequences of those traumatic events. For example, memories of childhood molestations or other traumas may suddenly begin to flood a parent's waking and sleeping hours and may impair present functioning.

As the parent reveals details of the events, children inevitably try to envision themselves in that parent's place during the trauma; this has been the case particularly with children of Holocaust survivors (Albeck, 1994). When children repeatedly and persistently imagine "the overwhelming scenes...without quickly escaping psychologically by changing the subject or denying its reality, psychological trauma may result."

These reimaginings and fantasies challenge the belief systems of the children and could potentially overwhelm them. The world is no longer benevolent and kind, just or controllable. It has no meaning, and they are no longer invulnerable (Janoff-Bulman, 1992). The traumatic event has secondarily shattered their assumptions about the world. They perceive that their survival is threatened and they experience disillusionment. A major task of therapy is to identify those beliefs and then, if indicated, work on belief change. Children's belief systems about safety, trust, power, esteem, and intimacy (McCann & Pearlman, 1990) are generally less solidified than those of adults and, hence, children are more likely to incorporate the traumas experienced by their parents into their inner worlds. This incorporation and introjection influences later development and may cause splitting, regression, or quick acceleration into "pseudo-adolescence" or "pseudo-adulthood."

In view of these impacts of parental trauma, where can children turn? Many therapists treat the trauma victim in isolation, without recognizing the impact upon the family and the important role of family members in healing. Herman (1992) noted that the decision whether or not to include the family in sessions and what should be shared or discussed in those sessions rests with the survivor. She does not envision the purpose of such sessions as family treatment. Instead, they are designed to "foster the survivor's recovery" and provide a "little bit of preventive education." However, it is this author's belief that if the family is not involved in the therapeutic process, denial of thoughts, emotions, somatizations, behaviors, and relationship issues is perpetuated. Family members, as well as survivors, need to talk about their perceptions of the traumatic event(s).

Controversy exists as to who should treat the children of the trauma survivor. Can the survivor's therapist also work with the children both individually and in family treatment? Can that therapist have individual sessions with the children in addition to seeing the trauma survivor as primary client? In the experience of this author, children are supportive, motivated to learn, and willing to work in therapy both on family and personal issues: the answers to those questions are in the affirmative.

Therapy sessions with secondary victims must be flexibly arranged to suit the presenting symptoms and the family circumstances. Ninety-minute to two-hour sessions may include individual time with the parental survivor, or with a child or children as well as couple work, family work, or dyadic work with a parent and child or children. While the trauma survivor does remain the primary client, an important aspect of treatment is to validate the right of secondary victims to have their experiences acknowledged and framed as secondary victimization (i.e., placed in the role of supporting the primary trauma victim [the parent] while, simultaneously, processing and dealing with their own reactions). Each and every family member may process the trauma in his or her own manner. While one member is primarily expressing avoidant symptoms, another may be experiencing intrusive thoughts and a third may be having sleep disorders and other somatic symptoms.

Course of Treatment

The course of treatment has four stages: encounter and education, exploration of trauma and its impact, empowerment through skill building, and evaluation and termination. Each of these stages encompasses a variety of techniques, themes, and strategies.

Stage 1. Encounter/Education

The major goals of the encounter/education stage are connection with family members, establishment of safety, initial diagnosis and assessment (which then becomes a continuing process), developing a framework, and education concerning the PTSD paradigm. During this stage, all family members may be asked to draw what Figley (1988) referred to as a "traumagram": a modification of a genogram that maps each individual member's history of traumatic events (Markowitz, 1991). The core of this stage is developing a therapeutic alliance with family members. This task is frequently much easier with secondary victims than it is with the survivor himself or herself.

As part of this process, the therapist identifies his or her roles and boundaries as well as the boundaries and purposes of the sessions. The therapist reiterates that the primary client continues to be the survivor and that no session will be allowed to revictimize that survivor. This is done in order to build a safety container around both therapist and family. Creation of a safe environment for the survivor and family is an arduous, thoughtful process that is designed to meet each client's needs. Treatment, as Parson (1988) noted, must help to develop the home as a place of sanctuarial safety from stress.

Safety building involves creating a safe setting, presenting the self (of the therapist) as safe both within and outside the therapeutic setting, establishing safety limits in the environment with family members and with the survivor toward others and toward self, and creating a safe process of therapy. These techniques are described in detail by Williams (1994).

A major component of this stage is education of family members. As Matsakis (1994) noted, reframing from the PTSD perspective depathologizes the survivor and helps to explain and eventually eliminate unwanted symptoms (Gotbaum, 1992). The diagnosis of PTSD needs to be shared with partner and children in an age-appropriate manner. Children as young as six are capable of understanding conceptualizations of trauma and can learn to modify personal responses to symptoms of post-traumatic reactions.

Children vary in their willingness to listen to and accept the PTSD paradigm. However, normalization of the diagnosis and provision of literature to everyone are extremely important. While information exists for partners, little has been written for children of trauma survivors. Some children see the PTSD diagnosis as explanatory and validating, while others view themselves as victims of that diagnosis. Acknowledging the reality of trauma and traumatic reactions changes the lives of all family members.

A secondary component of the initial stage of treatment is to assess the safety level of the family. How much violence is occurring? What amount of self-destructive behavior exists? Are parents exhibiting angry, raging outbursts that result in feelings of helplessness, fear, or like rage in other family members (Williams & Williams, 1987)? Does the parent ever view his or her children as the enemy or as representative of a group of abusers/victimizers? It is important for the therapist to help children identify the amount of time they are able to tolerate verbal harangues or non-physical attacks. Physical attacks by the parent or retaliatory attacks by partners or children are not to be tolerated. Safety contracts then must be established. The reaction of family members to potentially hostile outbursts needs to be planned and discussed in treatment. It is extremely important to help children develop ways to cope with hostility without resorting to physical violence or retaliation. At the same time, in individual therapy the therapist works with the parent to modify aggressive expressions of anger.

If the parent is actively acting out toward himself or herself, it is also necessary to develop a safety contract in this initial stage of therapy. In addition, the therapist may help the family to develop a triage plan for emergency situations (e.g., should the survivor become suicidal). Family members can learn to recognize "what works" to calm escalating situations. This stage of therapy corresponds to the development of basic beliefs of safety and trust.

Stage 2: Exploration of the Trauma and Its Impact on the Family

During the second stage of therapy, the parent reveals what he or she decides the family and others need to know about the trauma history, as he or she gets in touch with that history. Since many trauma memories are dissociated and amnestic, this process may be ongoing as new traumas surface. In the therapy setting, partner, survivor, parent, and children discuss the extent to which knowledge of the abuse is necessary for each to have, as well as the amount of "gore" the partner and children should endure. Children, in particular, should not be exposed to excessively gory details.

Learning the History

Do family members want to know the story of each and every trauma or abuse? If the parent is a victim of sexual child abuse, is the idea of that type of abuse revolting and unacceptable? Do family members believe that sexual abuse, let alone ritualized abuse, even exists? How comfortable are parents who are survivors of sexual abuse in teaching their children about prevention of abuse? Do they use themselves as examples of victims? The revelation of abuse or trauma history must be age appropriate, without inappropriate or too early exposure to a variety of details of sexuality.

As Mason (1990) noted, listening to the story of the parent helps family members understand what he or she "went through." Effective listening tells the parent that he or she is important and has value. If family members are not able to listen reflectively and effectively, the therapist may model and teach these skills. As Mason wrote, "Active listening is hard to learn but is worth every bit of effort."

It is important that the parent exercise extreme care and caution when sharing with others. She or he should tell only those who are trustworthy. It is also important for the parent to examine his or her motives for telling. What payoffs is he or she seeking? Does he or she want support or approval? How will sharing help others in the family to understand family dynamics? The therapist can assist the parent to tell those closest to him or her, while cautioning that he or she does not need to tell others outside of that close circle of intimates.

When parents tell children, it is important that those receiving the information not question the validity of the trauma. As therapist and family jointly discuss the trauma, it is also important that family members not try to force their personal ideas about the trauma upon the children. Both partner and children need to avoid telling them how to feel or how to act. At this point in time, parents who are survivors need belief and acceptance, support and compassion.

Integrating the experiences of the parent into the family is an important aspect of this stage of therapy. In other words, it is important for family members to discuss and recognize how the trauma has impacted their lives. During this stage of therapy, emotions are often released and losses are identified and grieved. It is the appropriate time for trusting relationships among family members to be solidified as parent and family members alike develop personal power. This stage is the core of the therapy process and builds social supportiveness (Gotbaum, 1992).

Self-disclosure is therefore encouraged during this phase of treatment. All family members are asked to reveal feelings, insights, and fears. The therapist assists in creating the context for open expression, within limits of non-blaming and non-denial. This stage is in essence a family debriefing. Framing of the story and its impact can lead to subsequent reframing and finding of meaning.

Children's Needs

In this stage of treatment, children need to discuss their reactions to what is being revealed or has been revealed. Children may feel betrayed, particularly if their parent has not previously revealed or recognized the existence of the trauma and its impact on them. Children, in particular, may resent the amount of time and energy the parent spends on healing rather than on the children (Dietz & Button, 1991b). Children need to grieve the loss of the previous (or previously perceived) relationship with the parent, if that relationship was more nurturing and more child-oriented. As the parent focuses on his or her healing, the needs of the child may need to be met by others and the child may need to be encouraged to seek having those needs met outside the home.

Acknowledging and identifying those needs of the children is addressed specifically during this stage of treatment. Satir (1967) noted that needy persons with emotional pain frequently seek out and find other needy, hurting persons as partners or friends. However, neither member then has the inner resources to meet his or her own needs, much less the needs of the other. If both parents are trauma survivors and one of them is healed, then the other may no longer be needed (in his or her original role) within the relationship.

Children have the right of refusal in becoming co-dependents. Parents, as they heal, also have the right to refuse to allow children to become co-dependent. The primary responsibility for self-healing rests with the parent, not with the child or the partner/spouse. It is important that children learn to say, "I cannot give any more of myself to you unless I get some of my own needs met." The parent may also say, "I need space to work on my issues; I need time alone."

The more mundane needs of daily family living must also be explored and dealt with. It may be essential for the parent to maintain employment if the family is to sustain itself financially. Bills, budgets, and everyday responsibilities cannot be ignored by the couple or the therapist. Family roles and family rules, as well as family beliefs about basic survival, need to be explicitly stated.

Emotional Impact

The emotional impact of the trauma on the family must also be explored during this phase of treatment. Children need to be given permission to express emotion within specified limits and boundaries. Children can be taught to label and name their feelings, identifying variations and nuances (Matsakis, in press). Their frustration and blame may erupt into angry outbursts or they may express their angry feelings passively. Anger work can help build more appropriate assertive responses. These children may be angry because the survivor "has put them through all this." Suddenly, their lives have been changed forever. They now have to be aware of triggers, flashbacks, and other trauma-related phenomena. They may consider themselves "victims of a victim." One individual wrote, "unwitting victim, innocent bystander, an onlooker suddenly wholly involved in the incident not by choice or disposition but by happenstance" (Williams, 1991). This feeling of deception and sandbagging may result in less than sympathetic reactions by those children. A major role of the therapist is to encourage them to express healthy anger in healthy ways. They can be encouraged to play sports, exercise, or practice learned self-defense.

Children may also feel great pain, including sadness and depression, particularly if that pain results from knowing that a loved one has known horrific experiences. Another goal of therapy is to help them develop less overprotective, appropriate empathic responses rather than sympathetic or oversolicitous ones.

Groups for children of survivors can play important roles at this stage of the healing process (Kaplan, 1994). Sharing of mutual concerns, emotions, and reactions to the traumas of family members can help to normalize those responses.

Children of survivors can learn symptom management techniques as well. They can be taught to view the traumatized family member as healing rather than a "looney tune" or "two bubbles off level," phrases this author has heard used by uneducated others. They can also be taught to recognize and avoid trigger words or situations. As Dietz and Button noted (1992), allies and partners (and children) can "be of tremendous help...by serving as healthy role models" (p. 16).

Stage 3: Empowerment and Skill Building

All children need to control their lives and feel empowered. While telling one's story helps to begin that empowerment, establishing bound-

aries and rules for relationships solidifies it and helps secondarily traumatized children build self-esteem. Social-skills training or psycho education, part of this stage of therapy, focuses more on presenting family
problems and taking concrete action (Harris, 1991). This aspect involves
teaching expressive skills, empathic skills, discussion and negotiation
skills, and conflict and problem-resolution skills. Figley (1989) added
that this type of therapeutic work helps the family develop a sense of
shared purpose, control, hope, and future orientation.

It is easier to cope with the long-term impact of trauma if the family
learns ways to manage tension and deal with the meaning of the
trauma. Catherall (1992) noted that therapists help family members
change their perspectives, reframe or strengthen healthy beliefs, or find
external causes or programs to support. Devoting oneself to a cause is
an excellent way to establish an external support system.

Establishing healing rituals within the family to facilitate the processing of emotions, experiences, and meanings is important. Healing rituals have seven common aspects:

1. They involve a symbolic reenactment or passive reminder of the
   specific trauma (the names on the Vietnam Memorial Wall, burn-
   ing a letter to a perpetrator) and the specific impact of the trauma
   on each individual family member. Public rituals already in existence may be considered.
2. They include a period of preparation and symbol making. Sym-
   bols signify what was lost or changed by the traumatic event and
   have before-and-after aspects.
3. They involve everyone in the family in specific ways through
   action taking and emotional expression. The actions symbolize
   both beginnings and endings.
4. They have a setting that is a physical reminder or memorial or
   may be an anniversary date.
5. They have intense transformatory power.
6. They include guides (e.g., therapists, shamans) as helpers.
7. They consider the ways each individual family deals with loss,
   emotion, transitions, holidays, and transformations and respect
   the family's coping style (Catherall, 1992).

The family also needs to learn to take time out to play and to be
intimate with one another in healthy ways. It is of extreme importance
that some semblance of normalcy remain in the child's life when his or
her assumptions of stability, invulnerability, and meaning have been

challenged. A family that uses humor, cooperates, and expresses emotions openly in non-blaming ways reduces demands on one another and reframes situations into more positive, growth-oriented Gestalts.

The therapist helps children (and spouses) develop new communication skills and rules for talking, asking questions, and expressing emotions. Practice within the therapeutic session, with the therapist serving as a role model, can help that development. Communication patterns within the family may have been dysfunctional. Teaching new methods of communication (e.g., the use of reflective listening and paraphrasing) can facilitate coping and encourage exchange of ideas, emotions, and beliefs (Gotbaum, 1992). As the traumatized parent heals, as the family develops more functional patterns of interaction, and as the secondarily traumatized children heal, needs of each and every member for nurturance will be met more appropriately, recognizing their developmental stages and building self-esteem. Children need to learn how to help in the family healing journey without becoming co-dependent. What can they do to lessen the burden on themselves as healing occurs? Suggestions concerning chores, care for siblings, and self care can be explored (Landry, 1991).

Parents may be encouraged by the therapist to share what is going on within the family with children's teachers. The school experience can be a refuge for children (Werner, 1990). A favorite teacher, counselor, school social worker, or coach can become a confidant, positive role model, and have a protective function in a child's life. A consistent school environment can become a safe place for children experiencing secondary effects of trauma (Garbarino, Dubrow, Kostelny & Pardo, 1992).

Intimacy and privacy issues need to be addressed, particularly if the parent (or parents) is (are) a survivor(s) of sexual child abuse. In this case, it is important to help family members identify beliefs about intimacy, perhaps through the use of a belief scale (Williams, 1990). It is often very difficult for trauma survivors to feel and express intimacy. Intimacy rests upon feelings of safety, trust, empowerment, and self-esteem. Unsuccessful attempts to initiate intimate contact with a survivor can cause frustration and extreme anger as well as feelings of helplessness and loss of control for children. Learning how to play as a couple and a family builds trust and intimacy. The therapist can help family members identify activities that would incorporate play into the family's routine. Going for walks, playing board games, having a picnic, going to the movies, or going out to eat allow family members to relate on a different level of intimacy and thereby empower themselves and build self-esteem.

As noted earlier, exposure to abreactions, flashbacks, and other intrusive aspects of reliving of a trauma impact children's beliefs about safety, trust, and personal power and restrict their abilities to be intimate or have positive self-esteem. It is extremely important for children as young as five and six to participate in family sessions to help them deal with the trauma history of their parent(s). For example, in sessions conducted by this author, young children have been taught to talk about their feelings, to recognize alters in parents with Dissociative Identity Disorder (DID), and to abrogate their responsibility for taking care of a "hurting" parent.

Stage 4: Evaluation, Integration, and Termination

A major focus of therapy of children who have experienced secondary trauma within their family is the healing of those children. Family members are included in that process at various times. When the parent has been the victim of severe, ongoing trauma that necessitates long-term therapy, there may be periods of time when work focuses primarily on parent issues. Children need to be included in this treatment decision and, should a crisis arise, need to have means to access the therapist. Secondary trauma reactions in children may be resolved prior to trauma resolution in the parent, and the child may terminate treatment prior to termination by the parent. It is always possible, however, that children who have resolved secondary traumatic reactions may reveal their own abusive experiences that have been perpetrated both within or outside the family. If the child reveals that the parent has molested him or her, that abuse must be reported to the appropriate authorities and the treatment of both child and parent has to be reexamined and reevaluated as to course, appropriateness of continuation, or transfer to another therapist.

Termination sessions with the child assess, and they reframe prior symptoms into what Figley (1988), adopting Horowitz's (1976) thesis, termed a healing theory. The healing theory needs to be accepted by the child (Peterson, Prout & Schwarz, 1992). Part of this work, as has been noted, involves finding meaning in the trauma, meaning that may be gained through social action or the finding of a mission (Herman, 1992). As Janoff-Bulman (1992) stated, "survivors (and their children) often transform the trauma into altruistic acts that provide some basis for meaning and value in their lives," such as volunteering at hotlines, participating in outreach projects such as the "Tears for the Children" (1991) sexual abuse survivors' handkerchief project, or changing a vocation to help other survivors. Janoff-Bulman (1992) also noted that post-trauma work includes "rebuilding a viable assumptive world...to make sense of...victimization" (p. 125).

As the family looks back over its healing journey, how does it conceptualize the lessons that the trauma has taught each member? Family members may determine whether or not there is a "redeeming" value in the suffering that each member has endured. The family may examine what understanding each family member has as to earlier and present behaviors, beliefs, or emotional responses as well as how family members depathologized the trauma. Family members may examine whether or not they have developed their own personal skills and competencies outside and within the family setting. They may also ask what types of future contingency plans need to be made, in case the family meets with new traumatic events or if new memories make themselves known. In addition, they may query how the process has helped family members reconsider what is important in life (e.g., the family becomes more important when faced with the death of a child or a spouse). A final evaluation of family roles, capacities, and modes of survival concludes this process. Children may have developed personal "Trauma Books" that have remained in the therapist's office. These books become the property of the child at termination.

SUGGESTIONS FOR PROFESSIONALS AND CONCLUSIONS

When children are kept in the dark and are not educated about trauma and the trauma history of a family member; when they are not included in therapy and integrated into the safe world of the trauma survivor; and when their own issues concerning power, intimacy, abuse, esteem, trust, and safety are not explored and treated, true healing for both the individual and the family system will not occur. Through appropriate treatment, families can build a new homeostasis, learn to renew themselves, restructure, and reorganize. Through development of affiliation within the family and with supportive others, through mental and emotional diversion and play, and through contact with others in similar situations, families can alleviate their emotional pain (Flach, 1988).

The ultimate goal of treatment is to build resilience. The resilient family, much like the resilient individual, recognizes its own innate strengths and is independent in patterns of thought and action. It allows for patterns of give and take and provides support when needed. Children are allowed to make independent decisions based on personal empowerment and control. Responsibility for self, rather than for others, is high. Resilient families provide support and positive affect to one another. They acknowledge individual perceptions, emotional expressions or beliefs, and allow open expression. They provide material assistance and information to members (Silver & Wortman, 1980). Resilient children have a wide range of interests and activities, communicate well, are committed to the continuation of the family unit, have insight into the cause and resolution of family problems, and face life with a sense of humor. Each child is able to tolerate distress, views himself or herself as a separate entity, feels competent, and solves problems creatively.

Werner (1984) identified four central characteristics that resilient children have in common:

1. An active, evocative approach toward solving life's problems
2. A tendency to perceive their experiences, even if painful, in a constructive way
3. The ability to gain positive attention from others
4. A strong ability to use faith to maintain a positive vision of the meaning of life

In addition, resilient children have both a strong social orientation and a strong sense of autonomy. They find a source of self-esteem and safe escape in hobbies and creative interests. They often engage in acts of helpfulness and caring and seek emotional support from persons outside their immediate family. The resilient family recognizes the need for a balance between structure and freedom at both external and internal levels. Family interactions are based on respect of self, privacy, and other boundaries. Roles shift as situations demand, and spontaneity is allowed (Flach, 1988). Anthony and Cohler (1987) added that resilient children have resilient, reassuring, encouraging, understanding parents who help them process secondary trauma. Losel and Bliessener (1990) similarly found that factors contributing to resilience in children include cognitive competence, self-confidence, an actively oriented coping stance and temperament, positive relationships with others, and the capacity to make sense of the world. Werner (1990) also recognized that most resilient children use school in a positive way.

Children of trauma survivors can play important roles in survivors' healing journeys. However, they also need treatment for their own secondary post-traumatic symptoms. Many therapists continue to treat the survivor in isolation and fail to acknowledge those needs of secondary victims. Recognition and acceptance of the secondary impact of a history of trauma on the family lead to a more inclusive treatment response. A therapist who works with partners and children as well as survivors must be flexible, creative, understand child development, be able to treat children with respect in an adult-like manner (where appropriate), and have a system-wide focus. That therapist can help family members recognize personal limits—when enough is enough— and can encourage family members to seek outside supports and interests when indicated.

Family work helps the secondarily traumatized child to feel safe. Through family-oriented therapy, children resolve their "own stuff" as it relates to the survivor's trauma. They learn to self-modulate and self-soothe, to set boundaries and develop hope, to listen with empathy, to touch in a non-sexual manner, and to support and care without feeling overly responsible or co-dependent. Children must be assisted to have patience and resilience to deal with the repeated hostility, anger, rejection, threats, and hurt that accompany their parents' battle with the immobilizing effects of PTSD. Appropriate, developmentally based, education that normalizes the traumatic response, that rests upon the PTSD paradigm as a systems theory, instills hope and states that neither they nor their parents are crazy. It recognizes that the trauma is the basis of the diagnosis and the healing process. The therapist who works with secondarily traumatized children therefore infuses hope into an evolving, changing, adapting family system that is more resilient, responsive, cohesive, and balanced.

As Herman (1992) noted, the resolution of trauma is never final and recovery is never complete; however, trauma-based lives can become more "ordinary" with healing. The following poem, written by the husband of a survivor of ritualistic abuse, attests to that healing (Wible, 1988).

To the Child Alone, Inside

A sense of loss,
   deep, unknown,
   swept up from within my soul
   and from deep dream spoke
   and awoke me to share
   a clear vision of

a childhoodless child's
life without innocence:
   a sense of loving
without love's return,
   a sense of caring
without a parent's care,
   a sense of being at total loss,
   abandonment,
   alone.
It's monumental emptiness,
   like a darkened room,
   enwrapped my heart
   until a silent scream
   filled my bones with this
   childhoodless child's
   terror, real and stark.

Few moments from another's past
   have ever leapt inside my soul
   but all these memories must have crossed
   between us in a second's flash
   for it came not just from your story told
   but from our touching soul to soul.

And so late this night I write alone,
   write to free-up my shattered-self
   by recalling back of the innocence of
   the childhood that was my own
   and from those abundant stores
   share large parts of my comforts known,
   bring out of memory my childhood past
   and set them before this abandoned child
   that haunts my dreams, my heart, my soul.

Then let them together play,
   my child within and this childhoodless child;
safe, alive within my memories' home
   until the silent screams at last subside
and the terrors deep that welled-up inside
   flee at last this abandoned soul
that so comforted comes at last
   to peace and love and to be at one
   with my own childhood's soul.

REFERENCES

Ackerman, R.J. (1983). *Children of alcoholics: A guidebook for educators, therapists, and parents (2nd Ed.).* Holmes Beach, FL: Learning Publications.

Albeck, J.H. (1994). Generational consequences of trauma: A second generation perspective. In M.B. Williams & J.F. Sommer, Jr. (Eds.). *Handbook of posttraumatic therapy.* Westport, CT: Greenwood Publishing Group.

Alessi, J.L., & Hearn, K. (1984). *Group treatment for children in shelters for battered women.* In A.R. Roberts (Ed.). Battered woman and their families. New York: Springer Publishing Company.

Alexander, D.W. (1993). *It happened in autumn.* Huntington, NY: Bureau for At-Risk Youth.

Alexander, D.W. (1993). *The way I feel.* Huntington, NY: Bureau for At-Risk Youth.

Alexander, D.W. (1993). *When I remember.* Huntington, NY: Bureau for At-Risk Youth.

Alexander, D.W. (1992). *All my feelings.* Huntington, NY: Bureau for At-Risk Youth.

Alexander, D.W. (1992). *It happened to me.* Huntington, NY: Bureau for At-Risk Youth.

Alexander, D.W. (1992). *The world I see.* Huntington, NY: Bureau for At-Risk Youth.

Ammerman, R.T., & Hersen, M. (Eds.) (1990). *Treatment of family violence.* New York: John Wiley & Sons.

Anthony, E., & Cohler, B. (Eds.) (1987). *The invulnerable child.* New York: Guilford Press.

Barnett, E.R., Pittman, C.B., Ragan, C.K., & Salus, M.L. (1980). *Family Violence: Intervention Strategies.* Washington, D.C.: Government Printing Office.

Beckman, R. (1990). *Children who grieve: A manual for conducting support groups.* Holmes Beach, FL: Learning Publications.

Bell, C. (1991, September). *Traumatic stress and children in danger. Journal of Health Care for the Poor and Underserved, 2*(1), 175–188.

Black, D., & Kaplan, T. (1988). Father kills mother: Issues and problems encountered by a child psychiatric team. *British Journal of Psychiatry, 153,* 624–630.

Brenner, A. (1984). *Helping children cope with stress.* New York: D.C.-Heath & Company.

Briere, J., & Runtz, M. (1987). *A brief measure of victimization effects: The trauma symptom checklist* (TSC-33). Durham, NH: Paper Presentation. Third National Family Violence Research Conference.

Burke, J.D., Borus, J.F., Burnes, B.J., Millstein, K.H., & Beasley, M.C. (1982). Changes in children's behavior after a natural disaster. *Am. J. Psychiatry, 139,* 1010–1014.

Buscaglia, L. (1982). *The fall of Freddie the Leaf.* Thorofare, NJ: Charles B. Slack, Inc.

Carroll, E.M., Foy, D.W., Cannon, B.J., & Zweir, G. (1991). Assessment issues involving the families of trauma victims. *Journal of Traumatic Stress, 4*(1), 25–40.

Catherall, D.R. (1992). *Back from the brink: A family guide to overcoming traumatic stress.* New York: Bantam Books.

Davidson, J., & Smith, R. (1990). Traumatic experiences in psychiatric outpatients. *Journal of Traumatic Stress 3*(3), 459–475.

Davis, L. (1991). *Allies in healing: When the person you love was sexually abused as a child.* New York: Harper Collins Publishers.

DeAngelis, T. (1992, September). Children's reactons to war are examined. *Monitor,* 3233.

Depaola, T. (1973). *Nana upstairs and Nana downstairs.* New York: G.P. Putnam's Sons.

Derogatis, L.R., & Spencer, P.M. (1982). *The brief symptom inventory (BSI): Administration, scoring and procedures manual-I.* Baltimore, MD: Johns-Hopkins University.

Dietz, A., & Button, B. (1992). The challenge of survivors of childhood sexual abuse in adult relationships. *Treating abuse today, 2*(1), 14–17.

Dietz, A., & Button, B. (1991a). The challenge of survivors of childhood sexual abuse in adult relationships: Managing disclosure and confrontation: Family of origin, friends and associates. *Treating abuse today, (1),* 4, 26–31.

Dietz, A., & Button, B. (1991b). Reactions by Partners and Allies. *Treating abuse today* (July/August), 11–13.

Dubrow, N., & Garbarino, J. (1989, Jan-Feb). Living in a war zone: Mothers and young children in a public housing development. *Child Welfare, LXVIII* (1).

Erickson, E.H. (1967). Identity and the life cycle. *Psychological Issues, 1* (1, Whole Issue).

Erickson, E.H. (1963). *Childhood and Society.* New York: Norton & Company.

Eth, S., & Pynoos, R.S. (1985a). Psychiatric interventions with children traumatized by violence. In D.H. Schetky & E.P. Benedek (Eds). *Emerging issues in child psychiatry and the law* (pp. 285–309).

Eth, S., & Pynoos, R.S. (1985b). Interaction of trauma and grief in childhood. In S. Eth & R. Pynoos (Eds.). Post-traumatic stress disorder in children (pp. 169–186). Washington, D.C.: American Psychiatric Press.

Fields, R. (1989). Children of the Intifada. *Migration World XVII.* (3/4), 12–19.

Flach, F. (1988). *Resilience: Discovering a new strength at times of stress.* New York: Fawcett Columbine.

Figley, C.R. (1983). Catastrophe: An overview of family reactions. In C.R. Figley & H.I. McCubbin (Eds.). *Stress and the family: Vol. 2. Coping with catastrophe.* New York: Brunner/Mazel.

Figley, C.R. (1989). *Treating stress in families.* New York: Brunner/Mazel.

Frederick, C. (1985). Children traumatized by catastrophic situations. In J. Laube & S. A. Murdock (Eds.). *Perspectives on disaster recovery* (pp. 110–130). Norwalk, CN: Appleton-Century-Crofts.

Garbarino, J., Dubrow, N., Kosteiny, K., & Pardo, C. (1992). *Children in danger: Coping with the consequences of community violence.* San Francisco, CA: Jossey-Bass Publishers.

Garbarino, J., Kosteiny, K., & Dubrow, N. (1991). *No place to be a child: Growing up in a war zone.* Lexington, MA: Lexington Books.

Gil, E. (1992). *Outgrowing the pain together: A book for spouses and partners of adults abused as children.* New York: Dell Books.

Giovacchini, P.L. (1989). *Countertransference triumphs and tragedies*. Northvale, N.J.: Jason Aaronson.

Gotbaum, M. (1992). *Post traumatic stress disorder and family therapy*. San Diego, CA: IATC Conference Presentation.

Graber, K. (1991). *A ghost in the bedroom: A guide for partners of incest survivors*. Deerfield Beach, FL: Health Communications.

Green, B.L., Korol, M., Grace, M.C., Vary, M.G., Leonard, A.C., Gleser, G.C., & Smitson-Cohen, S. (1991, November). Children and disaster: Age, gender and parental effects on PTSD symptoms. *J. Am. Acad. Child Adolesc. Psychiatry, 30*(6), 945–951.

Hannaford, M.J., & Popkin, M. (1992). *Windows: Healing and helping through loss*. Atlanta, GA: Active Parenting, Inc.

Hansen, P.A. (1992). *Survivors and partners: Healing the relationships of sexual abuse survivors*. Longmont, CO: Heron Hill Publishing Company.

Harris, C.J. (1991). A family crisis-intervention model for the treatment of post-traumatic stress reaction. *Journal of Traumatic Stress, 4*(2), 195–207.

Herman, J.L. (1992). *Trauma and recovery*. New York: Basic Books.

Herman, J., Russell, D., & Trocki, K. (1986, October). Long-term effects of incestuous abuse in childhood. *American Journal of Psychiatry, 143*(10), 1293–1296.

Hindman, J. (1989). *Just before dawn*. Ontario, OR: Alexandria Associates.

Horowitz, M.J. (1976). *Stress response syndrome*. New York: Jason Aaronson.

Horowitz, M.J., Wilner, N., & Alvarez, W. (1979). Impact of events scale: A measure of subjective stress. *Psychosomatic Medicine, 41* (209–218).

Horowitz, M.J., Wilner, M., Kalatreider, N., & Alvarez, W. (1980). Signs and symptoms of post-traumatic stress disosrder. *Archives Gen. Psychiatry 37*, 85–92.

Jaffe, P., Wilson, S., & Wolfe, D.A. (1986). Promoting changes in attitudes and understanding of conflict resolution among child victims of family violence. *Canadian Journal of Behavioral Science, 18*, 356–366.

James, B.L. (1994). Longterm treatment of children with a severe trauma history. In M.B. Williams & J.F. Sommer, Jr. (Eds.). *Handbook of post-traumatic therapy*. Westport, CN: Greenwood Publishing Group.

Janoff-Bulman, R. (1992). *Shattered assumption: Towards a new psychology of trauma*. New York: The Free Press.

Johnson, K. (1989). *Trauma in the lives of children: Crisis and stress management techniques for teachers, counselors, and student service professionals*. Claremont, CA: Hunter House.

Johnson, S.W., & Maile, L.J. (1987). *Suicide and the schools: A handbook for prevention, intervention and rehabilitation*. Springfield, IL: Charles C. Thomas.

Kaplan, W. (1964). Treatment of partners of F. Sommer, Jr. (Eds). *Handbook of post-traumatic therapy*. Westport, CT: Greenwood Publishing Group.

Kehayan, A. (1990). *Self-awareness growth experiences*. Rolling Hills Estates, CA: Jalmar Press.

Kulka, R.A., Schlenger, W.E., Fairbank, J.A., Hough, R.L., Jordan, B.K., Marmar, C.R., & Weiss, D.S. (1991). *Trauma and the Vietnam war generation: Report of findings from the Vietnam Veterans Readjustment Study*. NY: Brunner/Mazel.

Lagario, J. (1991). *The life-cycle eduction manual.* Solana Beach, CA: Empowerment in Action.

Landy, L. (1988). *Child support (through small group counseling).* Mount Dora, FL: Kids Rights.

Landry, D.B. (1991). *Family fallout: A handbook for families of adult sexual abuse survivors.* Orwell, VT: The Safer Society Press.

Losel, F., & Bliessener, T. (1990). Resilience in adolescence: A study on the generalizability of protective factors. In K. Hurrelmann & F. Losel (Eds.). *Health hazards in adolescence.* New York: Walter de Gruyter.

Malchiodi, C. (1990). *Breaking the silence: Art therapy with children from violent homes.* New York: Brunner/Mazel.

Maltz, W., & Holman, R. (1988). *Incest and sexuality: A guide to understanding and healing.* Lexington, MA: Lexington Books.

Markowitz, L.M. (1991). After the trauma. The *Family Therapy Networker, 15*(6), 32–37.

Mason, P.H.C. (1990). *Recovering from the war: A woman's guide to helping your Vietnam vet, your family and yourself.* New York: Penguin Books, U.S.A.

Matsakis, A. (1989). Dual trauma couples. *Vet Center Voice 10*(6), 3–5.

Matsakis, A. (1994). Dual, triple, and quadruple trauma couples: Dynamics and treatment issues. In M.B. Williams & J.F. Sommer, Jr. (Eds.). *Handbook of post-traumatic therapy.* Westport, CT: Greenwood Publishing Group.

McCann, I.L., & Pearlman, L.A. (1990). *Psychological trauma and the adult survivor.* New York: Brunner/Mazel.

McCubbin, H., & Figley, C.R. (1983) Bridging normative and catastrophic family stress. In H.I. McCubbin & C.R. Figley (Eds.). *Stress and the family, Vol. 1: Coping with normative transitions.* New York: Brunner/Mazel.

McCubbin, M.A., & McCubbin, H.I. (1989). Theoretical orientations of family stress and coping. In C.R. Figley (Ed.). *Treating stress in families* (pp. 3–43). New York: Brunner/Mazel.

McNully, R.J. (1994). What stressors produce DSM III-R post traumatic stress disorder in children. In J. Davidson & E. Foa (Eds.). *Posttraumatic stress disorder in review: Recent research and future developments.* Washington, DC: American Psychiatric Press.

Murray, H.A., & Kluckhorn, C. (1953). Outline of a conception of peersonality. In C. Kluckhorn & H.A. Murray (Eds.). *Personality in nature, society, and culture (2nd Ed., Rev)* (pp. 3–49). New York: Alfred A. Knopf.

National Organization of Victims' Assistance (1990 July). *Syllabus: National Crisis Response Team Training Institute: Participant's Manual. Class 16: Children's reactions to trauma.* Washington, DC: Author.

Okun, B. (1984). Family therapy and the schools. In B. Okun (Ed.). *Family therapy with school related problems* (pp. 1–12). Rockville, MD: Aspen Publications.

Parson, E.R. (1988). Post-traumatic self disorders (PTsfD): Theoretical and practical considerations in psychotherapy of Vietnam war veterans. In J.P. Wilson, Z. Harel, & B. Kahana (Eds.). *Human adaptation to extreme stress: From the holocaust to Vietnam.* (pp. 245–283). New York: Plenum Press.

Pearlman, L., & McCann, I.L. (1994). Taking a trauma history. In M.B. Williams & J.F. Sommer, Jr. (Eds.). *Handbook of posttraumatic therapy.*Westport, CT: Greenwood Publishing Troup.

Peterson, K.C., Prout, M.F., & Schwarz, R. (1992). *Posttraumatic stress disorder: A clinician's guide.* Plenum Press: New York.

Pynoos, R., & Eth, S. (1986a). Witnessing violence: Special interventions with children. In M. Lystad (Ed.). *Violence and the family* (pp. 193–216). New York: Brunner/Mazel.

Pynoos, R., & Eth, S. (1986b). Witness to violence: The child interview: The child interview. *Journal of the American Academy of Child Psychiatry 25,* 306–319.

Pynoos, R., & Nader, K. (1988, October). Psychological first aid and treatment approach to children exposed to community violence: Research implications. *Journal of Traumatic Stress, 1*(4), 445–474.

Pynoos, R., Frederick, C., Nader, K., Arovo, E., Steinberg, A., Eth, S., Nunez, F., & Fairbanks, L. (1987). Life threat and post-traumatic stress in school age children. *Arch. Gen. Psychiatry, 44,* 1057–1063.

Richter, J. (1991). *Children and Violence.* Plenary Panel: Public Policy. Washington, D.C.: 7th Annual Meeting of the International Society for Traumatic Stress Studies.

Roberts, A.R. (1990). *Crisis intervention handbook: Assessment, treatment and research.* Belmont, CA: Wadsworth, Inc.

Roberts, A.R., & Roberts, B.S. (1990). A comprehensive model for crisis intervention with battered women and their children. In S. Stith, M.B. Williams, & K. Rosen (Eds.). *Violence hits home* (pp. 25–46). New York: Springer Publishing Company.

Rosenberg, M.S. (1987). Children of battered women: The effects of witnessing violence on their social problem-solving abilities. *Behavioral Therapist, 4,* 85–89.

Rosenheck, R. (1986). Impact of post-traumatic stress disorder of World War II on the next generation. *The Journal of Nervous and Mental Disease, 174*(6), 319–327.

Rosenheck, R., & Nathan, P. (1985). Secondary traumatization in children of Vietnam veterans. *Hospital and Community Psychiatry, 36*(5), 538–539.

Rosenthal, D., Sadler, A., & Edwards, W. (1987). Families and post-traumatic stress disorder. In D. Rosenthal (Ed.). *Family stress.* Rockville, MD: Aspen Publsihers, Inc.

Rutter, M. (1987). Continuyities and Discontinuities from infance. In J. Osofsky (Ed.). *Handbook of infant development.* New York: John Wiley & Sons.

Sameroff, A.J., Siefer, R., Barocas, R., Zax, M., & Greenspan, S. (1987). Intelligence quotient scores of 4-year-old children: Social-environmental risk factors. *Pediatrics, 79,* 343–350.

Satir, V. (1974). *Conjoint family therapy.* Palo Alto, CA: Science and Behavioral Books.

Selman, R. (1980). *The growth of interpersonal understanding: Developmental and clinical analysis.* New York: Academy Press.

Shirk, S.R. (Ed.). (1988) *Cognitive development and child psychotherapy*. NY: Plenum Publishing.

Sipprelle, R.C. (1992). A VET Center experience: Multievent trauma, delayed treatment type. In D.W. Foy (Ed.). *Treating PTSD: Cognitive-behavioral strategies* (pp. 13–18). New York: Guilford Press.

Silver, R.L., & Wortman, C.B. (1980). Coping with undesirable life events. In J. Garber and M.E.P. Seligman (Eds). *Human helplessness: Theory and application*. New York: Academic Press.

Slaby, A.E. (1989). *Aftershock: Surviving the delayed effects of trauma, crisis and loss*. New York: Villard Books.

Smith, S.M. (1983). Disaster: Family disruption in the wake of natural disaster. In C.R. Figley & H.I. McCubbin (Eds.). *Stress and the family, Vol. II. Coping with catastrophe*. New York: Brunner/Mazel.

Sommer, J.F. Jr. (June 1992). Personal interview.

Spear, J. (1988). *Handbook for husbands/partners of women who were sexually abused as children*. Ashland, OR: J. Spear.

Steele, W. (1992). *Preventing self destruction: A manual for school crisis response teams*. Holmes Beach, FL: Learning Publications.

Strauss, M.A., Gelles, R.J., & Steinmetz, S.K. (1980). *Behind closed doors: Violence in the American family*. Garden City, NY: Anchor Press/Doubleday.

Strauss, M.A., Gelles, R.J., & Steinmetz, S.K. (1981). *Behind closed doors: Violence in the American family*. Newbury Park, CA: Sage Publishing Company.

Tears for the Children (1992). Descriptive pamphlet.

Terr, L. (1979). Children of Chowchilla: Study of psychic trauma. *Psychoanaly, Stud, Child 34*, 547–623.

Terr, L. (1981). Forbidden games: Post-traumatic child's play. *Journal American Acad. Child Psychiatry, 20*, 741–760.

Terr, L. (1985). Children traumatized in small groups. In S. Eth & R. Pynoos (Eds.). *Post-traumatic stress disorder in children*. Washington, D.C.: American Psychiatric Press.

Terr, L. (1989). Treating psychic trauma in children. *Journal of Traumatic Stress, 2*(3), 3–20.

Terr, L. (1990a). *Too scared to cry*, New York: Harper & Row.

Terr, L. (1990b). *Children's responses* to the Challenger disaster. *Washington, D.C.: New Research Program and Abstracts Presentation*. 143rd Meeting, American Psychiatric Association.

Terr, L. (1991). Childhood traumas: An outline and overview. *American Journal of Psychiatry, 148*,(1), 10–20.

Vondra, J.I. (1990). Sociological and ecological factors. In R.T. Ammerman & M. Hersen (Eds.). *Children at Risk: An evaluation of factors contributing to child abuse and neglect*. New York: Plenum Press.

Webb, N.B. (Ed.) (1992). *Play therapy for children in crisis: A casebook for practitioners*. New York: Brunner/Mazel.

Weinfeld, M., & Sigal, J.J. (1986). Knowledge of the Holocaust among adult children of survivors. *Canadian Ethnic Studies*, XVIII (1), 66–73.

Werner, E.E. (1984). Resilient children. *Young Children, 68–72.*

Werner, E.E. (1990). Protective factors and individual resilience. In, S.J. Miesel and J.P. Shonkoff (Eds.). *Handbook of early childhood education.* Cambridge, England: Cambridge University Press.

White, E.B. (1952). *Charlotte's web.* New York: Harper & Row.

Wible, R. (1988). *To the Child alone, inside.* Unpublished poem.

Williams, G. (1992). Children of the wall. *The American Legion, 132*(14), 30–31, 57.

Williams, M.B. (1990). *Post-traumatic stress disorder and child sexual abuse: The enduring effects.* Santa Barbara, CA: Unpublished doctoral dissertation.

Williams, M.B. (1991a). Clinical work with families of MPD patients: Assessment and issues for practice. *Dissociation, IV*(2), 92–98.

Williams, M.B. (1991b). *Williams-McPearl (TSI) Belief Scale.* Santa Barbara, CA: Unpublished dissertation research instrument.

Williams, M.B. (1994a). Intervention with child victims of trauma in the school setting. In M.B. Williams & J.F. Sommer, Jr. (Eds.). *Handbook of post-traumatic therapy.* Westport, CT: Greenwood Publishing Group.

Williams, M.B. (1994b). Establishing safety in survivors of servere abuse. In M.B. Williams & J.F. Sommer, Jr. (Eds.). *Handbook of post-traumatic therapy.* Westport, CT: Greenwood Publishing Group.

Williams, C.M., & Williams, T. (1987). Family therapy for Vietnam veterans. In T. Williams (Ed.). *Post-traumatic stress disorder: A handbook for clinicians* (pp. 221–231). Cincinnati, OH: Disabled American Veterans.

Williams, M.B., & Sommer, J.F. Jr. (1994). *Handbook of post-traumatic therapy.* Westport, CT: Greenwood Publishing Group.

Wilson, J.P., Smith, W.K., & Johnson, S.K. (1985). A comparative analysis of PTSD among survivor groups. In C.R. Figley (Ed.). *Trauma and its wake: The study and treatment of posttraumatic stress disorder* (pp. 142–172). New York: Brunner/Mazel.

Worden, J.W. (1991). *Grief counseling and grief therapy: A handbook for the mental health practioner (2nd Ed.).* New York: Springer Publishing Company.

TREATING TRAUMATIZED PARTNERS: PRODUCING SECONDARY SURVIVORS OF PTSD

6

Rory Remer, Ph.D.
Robert A. Ferguson, Ph.D.

INTRODUCTION

In this chapter, we address the treatment of secondary traumatic stress disorder (STSD) in the partners of trauma victims. First, the phenomena of STSD and secondary traumatic stress response (STSR) are briefly defined and related to the concepts of primary and secondary victimization. Second, a model of secondary survivor healing (R. Remer & Ferguson, 1992b, 1995), is presented and discussed. It is based on working with partners of sexual assault victims and related to P. Remer's (1984) model of primary survivors' healing process. Third, the interface between the two models/processes is examined, as well as its implications. Treatment interventions are presented and reviewed in light of both clinical experience and relevant research and are made along two dimensions: treatment goals (education, personal awareness/development, and skill acquisition) and therapeutic milieu (individual, conjoint, or group therapy). Finally, consideration is given to some specific,

1-57444-047-0/98/$0.00+$.50
© 1998 by CRC Press LLC

essential treatment issues: (1) alcohol/substance abuse, (2) preexisting pathology, (3) abusive partners, (4) individualizing approaches, (5) STSD primary victims, (6) helping vs. overinvolvement, (7) multiple therapeutic interventions, (8) impact on the therapist, and (9) balance between primary and secondary victim needs.

Trauma has a ripple effect. Not only are the victims themselves affected, but in many ways so are all those close to them. STSR, the natural consequent behaviors and emotions resulting from knowledge about a traumatizing event experienced by a significant other, is stress resulting from *helping or wanting to help* a traumatized person (Figley, 1992).

For each primary victim, there are numerous secondary victims—partners, children, parents, family, friends. When one considers the number of people touched directly and indirectly by the traumatic events, the magnitude of the problem becomes apparent.

With so many involved, it is surprising that so little has been done to help secondary victims. Only a few articles are concerned with this group. Most do not address the personal distress they suffer. Until recently, in fact, secondary victims have simply been viewed as the support system for the primary victim (e.g., Feinauer, 1982; Orzek, 1983; Rodkin, Hunt & Cowen, 1982). Whatever interventions have been suggested have been geared toward helping the secondary victim become more effective in facilitating the healing of the primary victim (e.g., Bass & Davis, 1988); few have been designed to help secondary victims learn to cope with and heal from their own afflictions.

In earlier articles, published elsewhere (R. Remer & Elliott, 1988a, 1988b; R. Remer & Ferguson, 1992a, 1992b, 1995) and within this volume and in *Compassion Fatigue*, an attempt has been made to rectify the situation. The plight of secondary victims has at last been fully recognized (Barnes, 1997a, 1997b; Beaton & Murphy, 1995; Catherall, 1995, 1997; Cerney, 1995; Dutton & Rubinstein, 1995; Figley, 1995, 1997; Gilbert, 1996; Harris, 1995; McCammon & Allison, 1995; Munroe et al., 1995; Pearlman & Saakvitne, 1995; Steinberg, 1997; Williams, 1997; Valent, 1995; Yassen, 1995) and the time has come to suggest ways of helping them confront their issues—those involving the primary victim as well as those uniquely their own.

This chapter focuses on the healing of partners—those in long-term, committed relationships with primary victims. Our aim is to suggest specific interventions on the basis of what has already been effective. We believe, however, that a theoretical structure is essential first, not only for grasping the rationale behind specific interventions but also, and perhaps more importantly, to make such interventions more adaptable to the unique exigencies encountered with each case.*

---

* From studies concerning Vietnam veterans and their wives, it is clear that a history of war-related trauma has a negative impact on marital adjustment and on the psychological well-being of both partners. As a group, veterans exposed to combat in Vietnam show significantly higher levels of marital disruption than Vietnam veterans who were not traumatized (Laufer & Gallops, 1985; Carroll, Rueger, Foy & Donahoe, 1985; DeFazio & Pascucci, 1984; Card, 1987). Women whose Vietnam veteran husbands were identified as suffering delayed stress are themselves more likely to experience symptoms of anxiety and depression (Smith-Schubert, 1985) as well as feelings of self-blame, low self-esteem, and of being cloistered and overprotected (Brown, 1984). Solomon (1988) reported similar findings in a review of the literature pertaining not only to Vietnam veterans but also Israeli war veterans and their families, and Pavalko and Elder (1990) reported higher rates of divorce for combat-experienced WWII veterans than for those who did not see combat.

Though much has been written about treatment of the veteran and his family system, little attention has been paid to the individual needs of the secondary survivor. Treatment approaches for the family and/or the secondary survivor as an individual include individual therapy for partners, couples therapy (Rosenheck & Thomson, 1986; Solomon, 1988), group couples therapy (Solomon, 1988), group therapy for partners (Rosenheck & Thomson, 1986; Moyer, 1988), and family therapy (Rosenheck & Thomson, 1986).

Among the specific goals of therapy are (a) trauma-related education (Rosenheck & Thomson, 1986; Coughlan & Parkin, 1987); (b) skills training, such as problem solving and relaxation (Solomon, 1988) assertiveness training (Solomon, 1988) and communication skills (Jurich, 1983) (c) awareness/self-assessment (Rosenheck & Thomson, 1986); and (d) social support (Solomon, Waysman & Mikulincer, 1990). Many of these treatment goals will be further discussed later in this chapter when we present a comprehensive model for treatment for all secondary survivors, regardless of the type of trauma.

The information presented in this chapter is based on extensive work with the partners of victims of incest and sexual assault. Most of these have been men. However, the findings related to war victims closely parallel those of studies addressing the impact of rape and sexual assault (McCann et al., 1988; R. Remer & Elliott, 1989; Whetsell, 1990). Accordingly, the suggestions made here will be generalized from our experience working with male partners of female survivors of sexual assault, as well as the limited research available on male partners of trauma victims. However logical such extensions may seem, empirical substantiation is as yet lacking. In addition, the comments should equally apply to other types of secondary victims—friends, children, other family members, therapists. Again, however, the adaptations must be made in light of the unique characteristics of each (particularly children of different age groups).

PRIMARY VICTIM/SURVIVOR HEALING PROCESS

An undeniable link exists between post-traumatic stress disorder (PTSD) and secondary traumatic stress disorder (STSD). While the focus of this chapter is secondary victimization, some discussion of primary traumatization is necessary in order to provide a context from which to intervene on behalf of the secondary victim.

McCann, Sakheim, and Abrahamson (1988) provide an extensive, concise review of the effects of primary victimization. One need only examine Table 6.1 to grasp the scope of what can occur.

According to McCann, Sakheim, and Abrahamson (1988), life experiences help create schemata which in turn lead to five areas of psychological adaptation (emotional, cognitive, biological, behavioral, and interpersonal) which in turn lead to new life experiences. These subsequent life experiences must be assimilated in one of two ways. Many times, they

Table 6.1   Psychological Reactions of Victims

Category	Reactions
Interpersonal	Sexuality problems Relationship problems Revictimization Victim becomes victimizer
Emotional	Fear, anxiety and intrusion Depression Anger Guilt and shame Self-esteem disturbances
Behavioral	Aggressive behavior Suicidal behavior Substance abuse Personality disorders Impaired social functioning
Cognitive	Perceptual disturbances
Biological	Somatic disturbances Physiological hyperarousal

Adapted from McCann, Sakheim, and Abrahamson (1988)

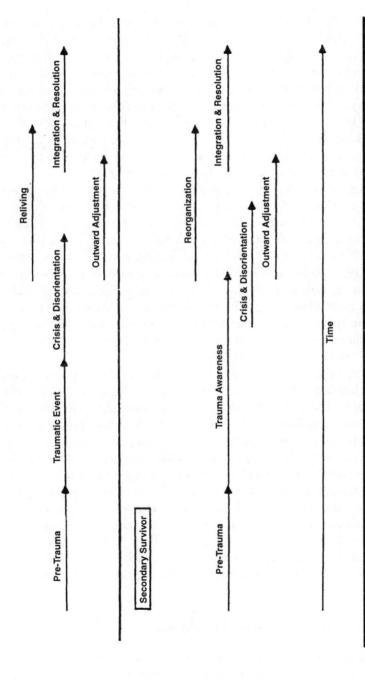

Figure 6.1 Similarities Between Models of the Healing Processes of PTSD and STSD Survivors; Adapted from Remer (1984); Worell and Remer (1992)

may be directly assimilated into existing schemata, the way someone could be "assimilated" into a familiar and comfortable piece of clothing. Another way for life experiences to be assimilated is for existing schemata to be altered or stretched to accommodate new and discordant information, just as a piece of clothing must be tailored to "accommodate" a different body. Keeping this theory in mind, and adding the perspective presented by P. Remer (1984) and Worell and P. Remer (1992) (see Figure 6.1), we have found a valuable viewpoint from which to operate when trying first to conceptualize the healing process of the primary victim, and then to build a model for the healing of STSD.

Implying that but one specific model has been developed to convey the healing process of every survivor would be misleading. Because each survivor is an individual, each will have a somewhat different healing process. In addition, the *type* of trauma suffered by the primary victim leads to variations in the general healing process. For example, Broadus (1992) found differences between survivors of trauma due to natural causes, human neglect, or human purposeful actions. Furthermore, Whetsell's (1990) study showed differences in the healing process for different types of sexual assault trauma. While acknowledging these potential differences, we feel there is a need for a general theory from which necessary variations can be produced.

P. Remer (1984) and Worell and P. Remer (1992) portray the rape survivor's healing process in six stages: (1) Pre-Rape, (2) Rape Event, (3) Crisis and Disorientation, (4) Outward Adjustment, (5) Reliving, and (6) Integration and Resolution. P. Remer's most unique and important contribution to the understanding of the healing process is the Pre-rape stage, which accounts for individual victim response differences by addressing such factors as cultural, familial, and personal history (e.g., sex role messages) and environmental influences (e.g., rape myths). Note the juxtaposition of the last four stages and, in particular, the final three, which are likely to overlap. Specific attention should be directed to the possible consequences of these overlaps. (See R. Remer [1990] for more details.) More extensive attention will be paid to this model and its use when educational interventions are discussed later.

A MODEL OF STSD AND HEALING

A theoretical/conceptual model for STSD and secondary victim/survivor healing has already been presented in Chapter 1 (Figley, 1997). Consistent with this formulation and integrated with that of P. Remer (1984)

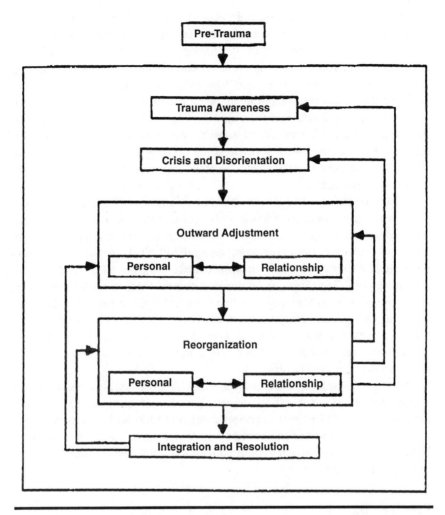

Figure 6.2   Flow Chart: Processional Stage Model of the Secondary Survivor Healing Process - Response to STSD

and Worell and P. Remer (1992), we briefly present the model (R. Remer & Ferguson, 1992b, 1995) on which our interventions are based (see Figure 6.1). While this portrayal is useful in seeing the necessary similarities between secondary and primary survivor healing, a subject addressed in depth later, Figure 6.2 is a better representation of the actual complexities inherent in the secondary trauma victim's individual healing process.

In many respects, the model posited here is similar to that developed by P. Remer (1984). Similarities are intentional and designed to capitalize on the strengths of P. Remer's (1984) model in order to provide as comprehensive a view of the secondary victim's healing process as is possible. It is also likened to P. Remer's (1984) model because the general adjustment in healing can be viewed similarly for both primary and secondary trauma victims. However, one important distinction should be noted: the primary survivor model focuses on intrapsychic healing—the interpersonal aspect is only implied. The secondary survivor model, perforce, must incorporate the interpersonal dimension explicitly.

While we believe the model is applicable to all STSD/PTSD relationships—parents, children, friends—our comments and observations are focused on partners, because the partner is usually the most directly involved and evidences the most generalized STSR. Adapting and expanding the model to apply to and include multiple STSD victims and systems is possible. Such an expansion would lead to many complexities, apparent from viewing just the "simple" dyadic situation. Dealing with the two-person circumstance, however, can be enlightening. Distinctions between the partner focus and a general STSD victim should become clearer as the model is applied in later sections, particularly in the conjoint therapy context.

As a processional stage model, ours is divided into six different stages (see Figure 6.1). The stages are: (1) Pre-Trauma, (2) Trauma Awareness, (3) Crisis and Disorientation, (4) Outward Adjustment, (5) Reorganization, and (6) Integration and Resolution. The first two stages happen in a linear fashion. The final four can, and almost inevitably do, overlap and recycle.

Pre-Trauma

As noted by Figley (1992), humans are social creatures and perceive their experiences within a social, as well as personal, context. Cultural belief systems, social role expectations, gender socialization, and other background influences greatly affect the psychosocial adjustment of survivors of traumatic events (Boehnlein, 1987). For example, some cultures (and many people in our culture) view anyone seeking outside support as weak or "sick"; conversely, they believe that anyone who is "well" should be able to handle his or her own problems, at "worst" only seeking help or support from within the family.

Barry was in his mid-thirties and working more than 60 hours a week to start a small construction business when his wife first told him about her childhood sexual abuse and said she wanted to seek professional help. The stress of self-employment, plus the fact that he came from a fairly incommunicative family, contributed to his initial reaction:

> In my family...we never talked about our problems, we solved them from within. And I guess I thought that's what she should do. When she wanted to consult a psychiatrist or psychologist about this problem, my immediate concern was cost. What's it going to cost? We need to weigh the benefits against the costs.

When Barry found out about a support group for men whose wives had been traumatized by sexual abuse, his traditional upbringing made him reluctant to participate.

> When I think of support groups I kind of think of Alcoholics Anonymous, you know, something like that or maybe a woman's type thing. I wouldn't think of that being a masculine thing.

In a sense, partners bring their entire histories to bear on the reactions to and understandings of another's trauma. If they are still struggling with their own self-esteem and identity issues, they may have difficulty meeting their own emotional needs, much less being a healing force in the life of the primary trauma survivor. Bradley, a retired engineer in therapy for his own dysfunctional childhood, struggled unsuccessfully to save his marriage to a woman with a history of childhood sexual abuse. He attributes the dissolution of the marriage, in part, to his own unresolved problems:

> I grew up with the idea that I could not succeed in anything. And I'm sure things were said. There was a horrible piece of verbal abuse. I was told at a very early age, I think maybe four or five, that they were really disappointed in me because they wanted a daughter. They had the room picked out and the colors picked out and the clothes picked out and then I was a boy. It had to have had a profound effect on me.

Context, environment, and prior learning are accounted for in this stage, just as they are in the case of the posttraumatic stress response (PTSR). In many instances, large portions of the backgrounds (schemata) of the primary and secondary victims will be shared. The more similar the two persons' histories—for example, being from the same ethnic background—the more likely it will be that their Pre-Trauma stages will be alike and often complementary.

Still, secondary victims may vary greatly in the extent to which they share a background with the primary victim. Previously unnoticed discrepancies in two persons' backgrounds may become apparent only after a trauma occurs. Such discrepancies, when they are great, cause problems in the coordination of primary and secondary survivor healing. The Pre-Trauma stage influences not only the flow of the healing process but also every subsequent stage.

Influence on the Pre-Trauma stage can be most easily effected through prevention (e.g., Yassen, 1995). Remediation, consisting of changing the schemata (Mounoud, 1976; Piaget, 1976), may be accomplished at a cognitive level, but significant impact on the emotional level may be extremely difficult since emotionally laden values and beliefs are targeted.

The influences of the Pre-Trauma stage, although pervasive and always present, may not be seen unless a significant stress occurs. When the trauma does occur, however, the effects of the Pre-Trauma stage will echo throughout the healing process.

Trauma Awareness

The Trauma Awareness stage may seem to be rather straightforward. It is not. How much and how soon secondary victims become aware of the primary victim's traumata depends greatly on primary victim healing (see Figure 6.3).

A short or long period may pass before the secondary victim becomes explicitly aware of the trauma, as illustrated by the contrasting stories of Jerry, a college student, and a middle-aged man named William:

> Jerry: I knew it before I dated her. I didn't know the extent of it until afterwards, but we were friends for about six months and so I knew a lot at that point.
> William: I was not aware of my wife's childhood sexual abuse until ten years ago. I'm 56—we've been married for 35 years. It wasn't until her mother's death that she even told me.

This time period may vary for a number of reasons: the primary victim may be loath to divulge the trauma or may remain unaware of the details or extent of the trauma or the secondary victim may not allow the extent or the details of the trauma into his or her awareness. And again, the Pre-Trauma stage may have significant influence on trauma awareness, including timing.

As more of the details of the trauma are learned and more of the effects of the trauma and the PTSR are felt, the Trauma Awareness stage may be revisited numerous times. Once the trauma enters the awareness of the secondary victim, a period of crisis and disorientation is experienced.

Crisis and Disorientation

Once the trauma is recognized, it must be faced and addressed. For some period of time, while accommodation, shock, denial, and confusion occur (Kubler-Ross, 1969; Piaget & Inhelder, 1969), the secondary victim will experience being off balance and out of touch. Length and degree of disorientation will depend on environmental, intrapsychic, and interpersonal factors, many of which will be directly related to pre-trauma experiences.

The relationship and both of its individual members may experience crisis and disorientation as a result of an immediate trauma or because of the emerging awareness of a trauma that occurred long ago. Therapy often precipitates traumatic memories that may create crises and disorientation before integration is eventually reached. Todd, a recovering alcoholic married to a survivor of childhood sexual abuse, describes how his wife's therapy affected him and the marital relationship:

> Prior to her therapy we had what I would consider a normal sex life. The more therapy [she] went through, of course she had to re-own her body and take control of her own actions, so of course, you'd get right up to the point and she'd say, "No, that's it, can't do it." And so it took me for an emotional ride.

Jerry, a college student, describes his personal disorientation resulting from witnessing his girlfriend's dissociative experiences:

> ...when I first started dating her and she had a flashback, I freaked out. I just didn't know what the hell I was doing and I was panicking.

The transference that therapists often encounter may also become an issue for the secondary survivor and contribute to crisis and disorientation. Again, Jerry:

> I feel sometimes like I've been placed in that role. I feel sometimes that she puts me in the role of the abuser and reacts to me as if I am one.

Outward Adjustment

Outward adjustment is necessary in order to marshal the resources of the secondary victim and of the relationship, so that both are ready to face the next stage of the healing process. Outward Adjustment, as the name implies, is often a brief, superficial return to what was the status quo prior to the traumatic event.

Outward adjustment for the secondary survivor may be based on denying the impact of learning about a significant other's traumatic experiences, as well as a sincere desire to be supportive to the primary trauma survivor. Mark, a graduate student in his late twenties, describes how his attempt at adjustment came at the expense of his own needs:

> It's like walking on eggshells. I'm constantly reacting to her. I'm taking her cues. Constantly being there for her. And I think that as a result I pretty much got burnt out because I don't feel that I got anything back. At times I used to wonder, "Am I some type of therapist, or what am I?"

After the immediate crisis, secondary victims often attempt to employ previously successful coping mechanisms; as a result, and to the extent these mechanisms are effective in this trauma situation, a period of seeming calm and normality may predominate.

Outward adjustment will occur on both personal and relationship levels. On the personal or intrapsychic tier, the individual defense mechanisms will dominate. On the relationship level, established role patterns will prevail. The two interact significantly, as indicated in Figures 6.2 and 6.3. Outward adjustment can continue for some time as long as *both* the personal and relationship aspects coordinate to maintain the veneer. Cultural imperatives, familial rules, or sex role socialization—Pre-Trauma stage expectations—will often support the temporary adjustment, particularly in closed systems. However, when significant change occurs to upset the homeostasis at *either* the personal or interpersonal level—most often some shift in the PTSD healing process (see Figure 6.3)—outward adjustment will disintegrate and the healing process will move into the next stage.

Reorganization

Reorganization also occurs at the same two levels, personal and relationship. As a result of the traumatic experience, new input must be integrated on both cognitive and emotional planes. On the personal (intrapsychic) level, the defenses that prevent the schemata involved from necessary adaptation will have to be addressed and overcome (McCann, Sakheim & Abrahamson, 1988); on the relationship level, new roles (interaction patterns) will have to be developed and implemented. To be effective, reorganization on the personal and relationship levels must be coordinated. Again, how difficult these changes will be is in part determined by the Pre-Trauma stage. The more flexible and resourceful the dyad and its members were prior to the trauma, the more effective and quick will be the reorganization. Flexibility and resourcefulness are the hallmarks of more effective and quicker reorganization.

When the parallel healing processes of the primary and secondary trauma survivors interface, it will hopefully lead to a positive reorganization of relationship dynamics, as described by 22-year-old Jerry:

> ...her abuse was not what first started changing how I looked at the world. It was her therapy and what she learned about having healthy relationships.

If reorganization is complete, at least for the particular level of trauma awareness, the healing process will move into the "final" stage. However, if the reorganization is only partially successful, it may lead to cycling back to one of the previous stages. If reorganization is successful but not complete, it may provoke further disclosures about the trauma. In an environment of increased trust, the primary victim may experience further trauma awareness; consequently, the awareness will be conveyed to the secondary survivor and the healing processes will cycle back to the Trauma Awareness stage for both types of survivors.

Unsuccessful reorganization resulting in retraumatization may trigger further reliving of the catastrophic event by the primary victim. This will again lead to further trauma awareness, which will have a negative effect on both the victims and their relationships. When reorganization is unsuccessful at the individual level, the relationship level, or both, another crisis is likely to be precipitated and the healing process will cycle back to the Crisis and Disorientation stage. Since reorganization takes a significant amount of personal and/or interpersonal energy, another period of Outward Adjustment will be needed. When enough resources are available to enable individuals to attain necessary intrapsychic change and to help members of a relationship realize the needed systemic change, reorganization can be achieved and eventually give way to the Integration and Resolution stage.

Integration and Resolution

Integration indicates having accepted the trauma and made it a part of the secondary survivor's personality structure at both a cognitive and emotional level. Resolution does not mean an end; it means the ability to see the ongoing aspects of the healing process and their continuance, perhaps forever. The secondary survivor must be prepared to continue the process indefinitely as new aspects of the PTSR are recognized.

Though young, Jerry has been with his girlfriend through much of her therapy and, like her, has managed to integrate the reality of the trauma into his own psyche as well as their relationship.

> Because I'm of the firm opinion that—and I even feel more so now than I did then—if you focus on the abuse, then that's going to be the focus of your relationship. The point is that the abuse did happen in the past and while you have to deal with it, it doesn't have to be the focus of the relationship.

Earlier in the healing process, new memories and insights usually throw the process back into Crisis and Disorientation. In contrast, new information during the Resolution and Integration stage is likely to lead the process back to the Reorganization stage, where the information is dealt with and worked through more quickly and effectively.

THE INTERFACE BETWEEN SECONDARY AND PRIMARY HEALING*

A distinguishing feature of STSD healing is dependence on information about and reaction to the healing from the PTSD. While the need for

---

* While not within the purview of this chapter, familiarity with a number of perspectives on interconnected processes would be useful to both practitioners and victims. For those not acquainted with them, most helpful are systems theory, role theory, and the concept of interdependence (see R. Remer, 1990).

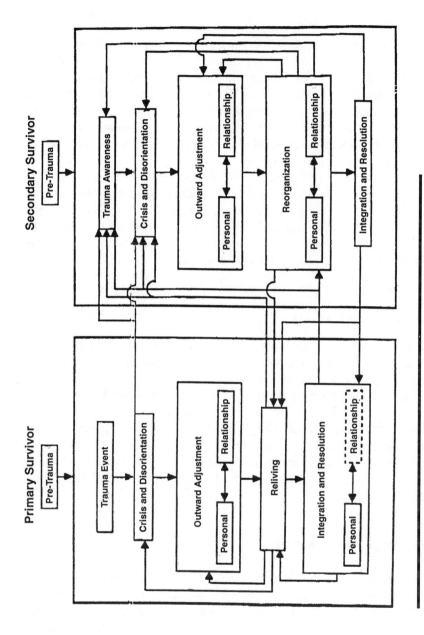

Figure 6.3   Interface Between the Models of PTSD and STSD Healing Processes

support makes the relationship aspect important in healing from PTSD, primary survivors must first focus on their own personal/intrapsychic healing. The explicit association, however, between the personal and interpersonal aspects of adjustment are often underemphasized for primary survivors (Bass & Davis, 1988). Secondary survivors, on the other hand, must attend not only to their own personal adjustment but also to the vicissitudes of the primary survivor's healing and to the impact of those shifts on the relationship. This statement is particularly true of partners of PTSD victims.

As is obvious from Figure 6.3, STSD and PTSD healing are inextricably intertwined. In addressing STSD healing, one of the main issues is how to mesh secondary and primary healing. Relational considerations—interplay, give and take, balance—are essential, not only for the resources to be available for healing of the primary survivor but also so that sufficient resources will be available for the adjustment of all those impacted.

Interface Implications

The PTSD victim is and must be the focal point of healing. Without giving primacy to primary victim healing, relationship healing will not occur or at best will be difficult to achieve.

If giving such primacy meant that the primary victim would have to heal completely before the healing of the secondary victims could begin, relationships would likely dissolve before healing could occur. Therapeutic intervention is usually necessary to support the healing of the secondary and primary victim simultaneously—to find a balance between both sets of needs, to mediate the interdependence of the healing processes.

TREATING PARTNERS

In approaching any therapeutic intervention, having a guiding structure in mind is invaluable. The structure we employ is based on the synthesis done by Egan (1975), who suggests three general stages to the therapy process: (1) understanding the problem from the client's perspective/building rapport, (2) extending the client's perspective, and (3) action. The structure suggested by Figley (1989) for working with traumatized families is similar. Figley views the flow of the therapeutic process in five phases: (1) building commitment to the therapeutic

		Treatment Goals		
		Education about Trauma	Awareness/ Personal Development	Skill Acquisition
Milieu	Individual Therapy	1	1/2	3
	Conjoint Therapy		3*	2
	Group Therapy	2	2/1	1

Figure 6.4   Schematic for Choice of Appropriate Therapeutic Intervention for STSD: Treatment Goals by Therapy Approach (numbers in cells indicate order of effectiveness: 1= most effective, 2= second most effective, 3= third most effective; * = conjoint therapy contraindicated except for recycling)

objectives, (2) framing the problem, (3) reframing the problem, (4) developing a healing theory, and (5) closure and preparedness.

One must be careful to remember, particularly in light of the labels "stages" and "phases," that the flow of therapy is hardly ever linear. A spiral is usually a better way to think about therapeutic progress. This element is recognized in the conceptualization of the partner's healing process outlined in Figure 6.2 and the interface suggested in Figure 6.3.

While the healing process, as portrayed previously, may eventuate on its own, the prospect is unlikely, at least in an efficient manner. Therapeutic intervention must be designed to facilitate movement through the various stages and preparation for self-determination.

In order to provide effective treatment within the context of strained resources and a large population of trauma survivors and their intimates, a two-dimensional model is proposed. The first dimension involves treatment goals. The second is therapeutic milieu (individual, couple, or group).

Treatment Goals

The primary objective is to help secondary survivors derive optimum support from themselves and the environment, thus attaining more individual satisfaction, while at the same time becoming more able to lend support to the primary survivor. This larger objective is accomplished by working toward three smaller goals: education about traumatic stress, acquisition of skills, and increased awareness/personal development. Although the goals of treatment will be discussed to suggest the order in which they are likely to be addressed, it should be understood that any particular client/therapist interaction may be different.

Therapeutic Milieu

The second dimension of this treatment model is therapeutic milieu, which refers to the approaches of individual therapy, conjoint (couples/ family) therapy, and group therapy. Each provides a different type of context and consequent impact, which can promote more effective and efficient intervention when employed appropriately at different stages of the healing process.

INTERVENTIONS

Services for each client, using the dimensions of Treatment Goals and Milieu, can be planned by referring to the schema offered in Figure 6.4. Which specific combinations (cells) would be used to describe treatment for each client would depend on a thorough assessment of the following resources:

- Time and personnel of service delivery organization
- Time and money available to client
- Cooperation of family members and friends
- Learning style of the client
- Motivation of client
- Pace at which client assimilates change

Education about Traumatic Stress

We have found that an educational component is indispensable in treating STSD. In a culture that perpetuates many myths about war and rape, two of the most common sources of trauma, the fact that so many secondary victims struggle with the conflict of blaming someone they love for the traumatic event is not surprising. Other misunderstandings also abound. "Why can't she just put this behind her?" is a frequently heard question. Assessing and addressing these beliefs is an imperative first step. In addition, secondary survivors clamor for any information that can aid in understanding. They want to know what their partners may be going through, what their own reactions might mean, and what they might be able to expect in the future.

This education is important for a number of reasons:

1. Those in the support network of survivors will cope better with some idea of what that person might be experiencing.
2. Network members who are integrally involved with the healing of their survivors usually want a basis from which to understand and to help.
3. Recognizing the parallels between the primary survivors' process and their own can provide a perspective for the complexities involved and can assist in understanding how the different processes are intertwined.

Familiarity by the therapist(s) with a specific model of healing from PTSD is essential if education is to be effective. We employ the model, mentioned earlier, developed by P. Remer (1984) and further presented in Worell and P. Remer (1992).

This model shares most of the salient aspects of other models (e.g., Burgess & Holstrom, 1979a, 1979b; Figley, 1985; Scurfield, 1985; Sutherland & Sherl, 1970). Because of its unique initial stages, however, it offers something more. Some of the differences resulting from various types of trauma can be anticipated without addressing each type specifically. In addition, it is a non-linear model that recognizes that adjacent stages are not mutually exclusive (see Figures 6.1 and 6.3). These overlaps allow the model to represent survivors' reality more accurately, a reality that is often characterized by complexity and confusion (see Figure 6.3).

Because of the possibility of confusion, defensiveness, and feelings of being overwhelmed, the learning style of the client is an important factor in determining the most effective and efficient method of providing information and challenging erroneous assumptions. There are many sources of information that could help uninformed or misinformed secondary survivors understand their partners' behavior, as well as their own reactions. Sources of information might include books, videos, lectures, classes, discussion groups, conferences, popular films, and survivor oriented organizations such as VOICES (Victims Of Incest Can Emerge Survivors) in Action, Inc.

Whereas one secondary survivor may only need to be directed toward a local bookstore to learn what is needed, another may do better in a discussion group that allows for interactive learning. Another client may be more story-oriented and learn more from films or television shows. Still another may need individualized personal instruction. Most would probably do best with some combination of the above sources. Again, it depends on matching the client's learning style with the optimum educational method. A ready list of possible resources should be the first element in the therapeutic assets.

The most effective milieu for the delivery of educational intervention depends on both the modality and the stage of the healing process. How an erroneous assumption is effectively challenged depends on finding a way to get the person to listen without becoming defensive. To whom, and under what circumstances, will the person be most open? If he or she is most open to the therapist, the individual milieu may serve best; if to the partner, then conjoint therapy is appropriate; if the person is more open to his or her peers, then the group therapy milieu may be most successful.

Awareness and Personal Development

For some secondary survivors, information about the effects of trauma on individuals and relationships may be all that is necessary. For many others, knowledge may help put much of the primary and secondary survivor's behavior into an understandable context but fall far short of addressing other individual and interpersonal needs. The denial that often accompanies trauma and its wake may need to be gradually lifted by facilitating deeper awareness of the personal impact. Whether secondary survivors and their relationships are characterized by confluence or isolation, any of the following phenomena may need to be brought into sharper focus: awareness of dysfunctional thought processes and erroneous assumptions; awareness of previously denied feelings, desires, sensations, and actions; and awareness of dysfunctional interpersonal dynamics such as boundary disturbances. As the clients become more aware, they will be better able to assess their own needs, as well as those of the primary survivors. Only by achieving a healthy balance between the needs of self and those of others can a secondary survivor offer support to a PTSD victim.

Awareness increases in two areas: trauma awareness and personal awareness. Concomitant with the increase in either type of awareness is usually severe personal discomfort typical of Crisis/Disorientation (Egan, 1975). Because many of the thoughts and feelings elicited— anger at the victim, desire to leave the relationship, self-blame, and so forth—may be unacceptable to the secondary victim, let alone others, an extremely "safe" milieu will be required to allow exploration. The STSD victim will need a non-judgmental, accepting ear. Conjoint therapy is *contraindicated* for dealing with this type of personal awareness. Sorting out which issues belong to which individual and which ones are part of the relationship is important. Given the usual *give and take* required of the partners involved in conjoint therapy, the demands are often too much to expect two confused, hurting individuals to handle. Neither can be fairly required to put his or her therapeutic needs second for the other's sake. The needs of the individuals and of the couple are better served, in the long run, by each partner initially receiving individual attention. As the cases of Jerry and Mark suggest, personal shortcomings and problems can be faced and appropriate ways to communicate functionally within the conjoint context can be learned. The primary victim cannot and should not be in the position either of being revictimized or of having to deal with these types of secondary victim struggles; the secondary victim should not be asked to do in therapy what he or she must do every day outside of it.

Group therapy can be helpful, particularly in latter stages of Reorganization and recycling through Crisis/Disorientation. Hearing others who have come to grips with the same issues and helping others with their struggles can be facilitative. Early in healing, however, commitment to group process may be difficult to secure. (We ask that group members attend at least five sessions, and if they decide to leave the group, they are required to say good-bye.)

Individual therapy is, therefore, usually the approach of choice. Building commitment to therapy goals and reframing the problem (Egan, 1975; Figley, 1989) can most effectively be accomplished in the context of a strong therapeutic alliance based on confidence in and comfort with the client/therapist relationship.

Both individual and conjoint approaches may be called for in addressing Trauma Awareness. Conjoint can be useful in promoting and supporting required memory reclaiming in a constructive way as the primary victim recycles through this stage of healing for a second or third time, or more. Individual therapy will be required in preparing the secondary victim to deal with the personal aspects. For partners more advanced with healing, group therapy may substitute adequately for the more personalized, focused individual therapy approach.

Skills

As partners gain awareness in any or all of the above areas, they are likely to recognize certain skill deficiencies as well. Many secondary survivor clients may lack the skills required to attend to their own needs, much less to be supportive of a traumatized partner. Others may be called upon to learn new skills that were previously unneeded. Skills such as communication, assertiveness, critical thinking, and supportive self-talk may be acquired in a number of ways.

For the sake of both efficiency and effectiveness, skills training can be most readily done in an interactive milieu. While the individual therapy context can be used, the group milieu provides both more resources and more support for such training. In addition, the benefits of vicarious learning, role reversal, and confidence built through multiple cognitive and behavioral rehearsals should not be understated.

In addressing the relationship dimensions (e.g., in Outward Adjustment and Reorganization) inherent in Figley's (1989) Preparedness Phase and Egan's (1975) Action Phase, group therapy is the first line of intervention. However, the transfer and generalization of relationship skills is likely to be enhanced by the use of conjoint therapy once both partners have healed and/or developed enough to approach the interaction constructively. Aiding both partners in the actual, gradual implementation of what may be a new mode of interaction is greatly facilitated through the guidance and control of the process by a skilled therapist.

TREATMENT ISSUES

A host of questions pertinent to optimal intervention suggest themselves: What are the positives and negatives to partners having therapists of the same/different gender? How long should the course of treatment be? Where can therapists get competent supervision? What impact does culture and/or gender have specifically? How can these and other factors be addressed most effectively? Treatment of STSD is such a nascent area that only a few empirically supported, directly generalizable answers exist. The best that can be done, at the moment, is to offer some clinical observations concerning some of the more relevant treatment issues encountered thus far.

Some secondary survivors may present more complicated or deeper problems or skill deficits. Through the process of trying to understand a partner's PTSR, some secondary survivors will regain traumatic memories of their own. Others will need to be treated for personality disorders. Others, upon realizing the difficulty and commitment often associated with changing individual behavior and relationship dynamics, will choose to abandon the process prematurely.

While many treatment issues arise during the course of any therapy, a number have become consistently manifest in our working with STSD partners. Awareness of these may serve to help in grounding the therapeutic work, if not in preventing the actual occurrence of difficulties.

Alcohol/Substance Abuse

In all too many instances, either the primary victim, the partner, or both have ongoing substance-abuse-related problems. While the substance abuser(s) may view the use of alcohol or drugs as a coping mechanism, secondary to or a result of the STSD, the abuse must be a paramount concern of the therapist. Most, if not all, interventions will be ineffective if the substance abuse is not stopped before other areas are addressed. Attending to this sphere first is so important that ascertaining the extent of any substance abuse problem should be included specifically in any evaluation/assessment/diagnosis. This stance may be at odds with the approaches suggested by others, including the view taken by other authors in this volume. Still, our own clinical experiences, those of many of our colleagues, and those of many other professionals dealing with substance abuse have indicated little, if any, lasting gain being achieved where any other course of intervention has been used.

Preexisting Pathology

Trauma is a stress situation. While the attendant stress will not necessarily create pathology, it will almost certainly exacerbate any present. In cases of severe Axis I or Axis II pathology, a therapist should be realistic about expectations regarding what can be accomplished given available resources. If severe pathology is suspected, a thorough, formal assessment will help the therapist decide whether or not treatment for PTSD and STSD is likely to yield success, and if so, what the actual duration of such treatment is likely to be. An inexperienced therapist may spend many unnecessary sessions concentrating on a trauma, primary or secondary, with a client whose preexisting pathology is so disturbing as to prevent the person from benefiting from such a focus. In such a case, an appropriate referral or consultation with other professionals is likely to be in the client's best interest.

Abusive Partners

A special case of preexisting pathology, and one specifically worth noting, is an abusive partner. Either the secondary victim or the primary victim may be the abuser (more often it is the male partner involved). Such instances, though rare in the context of STSD victims we see, are possible. Obviously, an abusive partner should not be considered part of the solution to this problem area but rather an obstacle to any possible healing. As in the case of substance abuse, the abuse issue must be separated and dealt with first. A dissolution of the relationship may be the only effective option available.

Individualizing Approaches

Certainly in conveying information, but also in other aspects of therapy, such considerations as learning style, cognitive ability, emotional maturity, interpersonal communication facility, etc. must be taken into account. For therapy to be effective, those receiving help must be met at their own levels, at least initially, before those levels can be changed. (This issue is an especially difficult one with which to deal in group therapy.)

STSD Primary Victims

More frequently than might be expected, STSD partners turn out to be victims themselves. In coping and working with primary victim partners, they are often triggered into remembering their own traumata. One way of explaining this phenomenon, which is also helpful in addressing it to some extent, is Bowen's (1972) concept of differentiation—people tend to couple with partners who match their level of differentiation and who complement them. Sometimes this leads to mutually supported pathologies.

Helping vs. Overinvolvement

Many effective secondary survivors are keenly aware of the impact of the trauma on both the primary survivor and the relationship. In fact, in many ways, they may be too attuned. A fine line often exists between helping (as a mode of personal therapy) and enabling (in the negative sense, i.e. supporting the pathology of the primary victim as a way of avoiding dealing with one's own personal problems). In many instances, because of the meshing of the two healing processes, clear boundaries are difficult to delineate or to maintain. STSD victims must be helped to learn to balance the needs and demands of the primary victim against their own, being neither selfish nor selfless.

Multiple Therapeutic Interventions

Actually, multiple therapeutic intervention raises not one but several important issues: (1) whether it should be done; (2) what the optimal combination is; (3) what the optimal distribution of labor is (e.g., who should do what assessment[s]); (4) whether there should be multiple therapists involved; (5) how efforts should/can be coordinated; (6) what the timing should be; and (7) how resources should be allocated, particularly if they are scarce. These issues often are related.

Unequivocally, multiple therapeutic intervention by multiple therapists is the optimal approach for this complex situation. Some combination of ongoing, continuing individual therapy for both partners, group therapy for both partners, couples therapy, and bibliotherapy will produce the best results in the most efficient manner. However, in most instances, such arrangements are not realistic. Victims have neither the time, nor the money, nor the energy necessary to make this plan possible (and that does not even take into account the extended STSD victim network). At a minimum, however, all these components should be employed at one time or another.

Given the intertwining of courses of therapy and the ever-present boundary issues, multiple therapist involvement, for both practical and ethical reasons, is indicated. Communication and coordination between therapists—which require legal "Release of Information" to be secured from both partners by all therapists involved—allow clients and therapists together to address the other attendant issues, openly and cooperatively, making necessary decisions and compromises in the best interests of all concerned.

Occasional conferences will facilitate the coordination of efforts. At the same time, the victims are provided with collaborative advocates at a stage when they may be needed. Consultations may also serve therapeutic value by modeling the type of interaction between and among participants that will be required of the partners. Demonstrating and teaching communication skills are essential, especially since other questions regarding distribution of resources have no standard answers and must be constantly negotiated in light of the conditions existing at a given moment. To be effective, however, the therapists must be aware of not only the boundary issues engendered by STSD for the victims but their own personal, professional, and theoretical boundary issues as well.

As noted, the optimal situation would be a balanced combination of individual, group, and conjoint therapy. However, reality dictates less. In most instances, group intervention is the approach of choice for secondary victims, because the system's resources are directed to the primary victim, and more external resources can be made available and shared in addressing the various demands of STSD healing in this milieu.

Impact on the Therapist

PTSD/STSD is a high "burnout" area. This problem has been addressed extensively in *Compassion Fatigue* (Beaton & Murphy, 1995; Catherall, 1995; Cerney, 1995; Dutton & Rubinstein, 1995; Figley, 1995; Harris, 1995; McCammon & Allison, 1995; Munroe et al., 1995; Pearlman & Saakvitne, 1995; Valent, 1995; Yassen, 1995).

No matter how experienced or how well trained therapists are, they must realize that the healing process will be arduous. Mistakes will be made and there will be moments of uncertainty. Because of the type of involvement required to foster STSD healing, therapists are also to be considered secondary survivors. As such, their resources are significantly taxed. Without self-awareness, as well as knowledge of STSD and PTSD, therapists can easily become secondary victims themselves. It is important to mention this issue within the context of treating partners because, all too often, therapist fail to strike the required balance themselves. As mentioned previously, the impact of modeling, either positive or negative, cannot be minimized.

Balance and Primary Victim Primacy

Far and away, the most pervasive issue in dealing with STSD victims is the question of the primacy of primary victim healing. Cognitively, emotionally, and behaviorally, secondary victims, even more than primary ones, are torn between their own needs and those of their partners.

Immediately following severe trauma, the primary victim will be in distress. At that time, the need for help is easily recognized. However, long after the trauma, primary victims may still be in trouble and, consequently, in need of support. Even the most "resourceful" person will be greatly stretched to cope without additional help.

At this point, two things must happen: (1) secondary victims must support and supply resources for the healing of the primary victim and (2) partners must not make demands on the resources of the primary victim. In the initial phases of healing, little if any reciprocity or balance can be expected in relationships. (This may also be the case during other particularly disturbing stages of healing, e.g., Reliving.)

When such instances occur, secondary victims must put some, if not all, of their competing needs aside to support the primary victim in whatever ways possible. Also, when secondary victims experience needs, they will have to look elsewhere for the resources to meet them. (However, addressing secondary victims' needs elsewhere may have to be suspended temporarily if, in the process of doing so, the healing of the primary victim, at least through the initial critical phases of the healing process, would be disrupted.)

In the long run, however, a return to some semblance of an interdependent pattern must occur. Reliance of the primary victim on the secondary victims to direct all resources of the support network to the primary victim cannot go on indefinitely. Inevitably relationships will break down if there is not some balance and some reciprocity restored (Henry, 1990). Dissolution may not be welcomed, but it may be the only viable option available if optimal healing is to occur for both partners.

The restoration of the balance or the establishment of a new balance may demand therapeutic intervention and usually does. New methods of negotiating the give and take in the relationship may be required. In fact, given that the healing process of both primary and secondary victims will be ongoing for a long period, if not for a lifetime, there should be no expectation that the original relationship patterns can be functionally reestablished. Expectations should be that new, more effective patterns will have to be implemented in the place of the old.

For example, the primary victim may have to learn to function in the role of "taker" instead of that of "giver" (i.e., in the role of one being emotionally supported and dependent instead of the role of one strong and independent). These transitions may be particularly difficult to affect if Pre-Trauma stage influences interfere (e.g., if sex role socialization or cultural rules have contributed to inflexibility in the role patterns). Overall, however, both secondary and primary victims may benefit a great deal from the increase in role flexibility required to initiate Integration and Resolution, continued and continual healing. In fact, the sense of "coupleness" engendered by overcoming a difficult situation together and the power derived from becoming more effective, healthier individuals can generalize to, and even pervade, other relationships and other areas of life.

SUMMARY AND CONCLUSION

STSD (secondary victim) healing depends on that of the primary victim; primary victim healing depends on the resources and support available in the social system. Without recognizing the interplay in these healing processes, successful healing of each partner and the relationship is improbable. If some healing does occur, it may come at someone's expense, most likely that of the secondary victim. Therapeutic support is essential.

Even with therapeutic support, there is no guarantee that either the partners or their relationships will survive intact. Major revisions in personal constitution and in the patterns of relationships will be required.

The healing and therapeutic processes of the secondary victim are obviously involved with and subject to the therapy and healing of the primary victim. Still, as much as STSD healing is dependent on the healing of the primary victim, primary victim healing also relies on that of the partner. If secondary victims do not become secondary survivors, fewer resources will be available to support the healing of the primary victim. The processes so significantly intertwine that the production of a tapestry of healing requires the deft touch of an expert weaver to achieve a viable, coherent pattern. But the satisfaction for all involved from having repaired the damaged fabric, or even better, having created a new, more vibrant pattern, is well worth the effort demanded.

When the myriad problems, complexities, and challenges have been met effectively, the partners and the partnership emerge stronger, healthier, and more adept. Often the social support networks involved are expanded and enhanced, both as a result of more open contact with others coping with the same problems and as a consequence of the development of better communication skills. The sense of accomplishment, and consequent empowerment may lead to a fuller, more fruitful, joyous existence than might have ever before been imagined, let alone expected.

REFERENCES

Barnes, M. (1997a). Understanding the secondary traumatic stress of parents. In C. Figley (Ed.), *Burnout in families: The systemic costs of caring*. Boca Raton, FL: St. Lucie Press.

Barnes, M. (1997b). Treating burnout in families following childhood trauma. In C. Figley (Ed.), *Burnout in families: The systemic costs of caring*. Boca Raton, FL: St. Lucie Press.

Bass, E., & Davis, L. (1988). *The courage to heal: A guide for women survivors of child sexual abuse*. New York: Harper and Row.

Beaton, R., & Murphy, S. (1995). Working with people in crisis: Research implications. In C. Figley (Ed.), *Compassion fatigue: Coping with secondary traumatic stress disorder in those who treat the traumatized* (pp. 51–81). New York: Brunner/Mazel.

Boehnlein, J.K. (1987). Culture and society in post traumatic stress disorder: Implications for psychotherapy. *American Journal of Psychiatry, 41,* 519–513.

Bowen, M. (1972). Toward the differentiation of a self in one's own family. In J. Framo (Ed.), *Family interaction: A dialogue between family researchers and family therapists* (pp. 175–200). New York: Springer.

Broadus, M.J. (1992). *The influence of the nature of the event, gender and gender schemata on the long-term effects of traumatization*. Unpublished doctoral dissertation. Lexington: University of Kentucky.

Brown, P.C. (1984). Legacies of a war: Treatment considerations with Vietnam veterans and their families. *Social Work, 29,* 372–379.

Burgess, A.W., & Holmstrom, L.L. (1979a). Adaptive strategies and recovery from rape. *American Journal of Psychiatry, 136,* 1278–1282.

Burgess, A.W., & Holstrom, L.L. (1979a). *Rape: Crisis and recovery*. Bowie, MD: Robert J. Brady.

Card, J.J. (1987). Epidemiology of PTSD in a national cohort of Vietnam veterans. *Journal of Clinical Psychology, 43,* 6–17.

Carroll, E.M., Rueger, D.B., Foy, D.W., & Donahoe, C.P. (1985). Vietnam combat veterans with posttraumatic stress disorder: Analysis of marital and cohabitating adjustment. *Journal of Abnormal Psychology, 94,* 329–337.

Catherall, D. (1995). Preventing institutional secondary traumatic stress disorder. In C. Figley (Ed.), *Compassion fatigue: Coping with secondary traumatic stress disorder in those who treat the traumatized* (pp. 232–248). New York: Brunner/ Mazel.

Catherall, D. (1997). Treating traumatized families. In C. Figley (Ed.), *Burnout in families: The systemic costs of caring*. Boca Raton, FL: St. Lucie Press.

Cerney, M.S. (1995). Treating the "heroic treaters." In C. Figley (Ed.), *Compassion fatigue: Coping with secondary traumatic stress disorder in those who treat the traumatized* (pp. 131–149). New York: Brunner/Mazel.

Coughlan, K., & Parkin, C. (1987). Woman partners of Vietnam vets. *Journal of Psychosocial Nursing and Mental Health Services, 25*(10), 25–27.

DeFazio, V.J., & Pascucci, N.J. (1984). Return to Ithaca: A perspective on marriage and love in post traumatic stress disorder. *Journal of Contemporary Psychotherapy, 14*, 76–89.

Dutton, M.A., & Rubinstein, F.L. (1995). Working with people with PTSD: Research implications. In C. Figley (Ed.), *Compassion fatigue: Coping with secondary traumatic stress disorder in those who treat the traumatized* (pp. 82–100). New York: Brunner/Mazel.

Egan, G. (1975). *The skilled helper: A model for systematic helping and personal relating*. Monterey, CA: Brooks/Cole Publishing.

Feinauer, L. (1982). Rape: A family crisis. *American Journal of Family Therapy, 10*(4), 35–39.

Figley, C.R. (1985). From victim to survivor: Social responsibility in the wake of catastrophe. In C.R. Figley (Ed.), *Trauma and its wake: The study and treatment of post traumatic stress disorder* (pp. 398–415). New York: Brunner/ Mazel.

Figley, C.R. (1989). *Helping traumatized families*. San Francisco: Jossey-Bass.

Figley, C.R. (1992). Traumatic stress reactions and disorders: Reconfiguring PTSD. Paper presented to a Special Panel on DSMIV at the ISTSS World Conference, Amsterdam, Holland, June 24.

Figley, C.R. (1995). Compassion fatigue as a secondary traumatic stress disorder: An overview. In C. Figley (Ed.), *Compassion fatigue: Coping with secondary traumatic stress disorder in those who treat the traumatized* (pp. 1–20). New York: Brunner/Mazel.

Figley, C.R. (1997). Burnout as systemic traumatic stress: A model for helping traumatized families. In C. Figley (Ed.), *Burnout in families: The systemic costs of caring*. Boca Raton, FL: St. Lucie Press.

Gilbert, K. (1997). Understanding the secondary traumatic stress of spouses. In C. Figley (Ed.), *Burnout in families: The systemic costs of caring*. Boca Raton, FL: St. Lucie Press.

Harris, C.J. (1995). Sensory-based therapy for crisis counselors. In C. Figley (Ed.), *Compassion fatigue: Coping with secondary traumatic stress disorder in those who treat the traumatized* (pp. 101–114). New York: Brunner/Mazel.

Henry, S. (1990). Can a marriage survive tragedy? *Parade Magazine*, July 15, 4–6.

Jurich, A.P. (1983). The Saigon of the family's mind: Family therapy with families of Vietnam veterans. *Journal of Marital and Family Therapy, 9*, 355–363.

Kubler-Ross, E. (1969). *On death and dying.* New York: McMillan.

Laufer, R.S., & Gallops, M.S. (1985). Life-course effects of Vietnam combat and abusive violence: Marital patterns. *Journal of Marriage and the Family, 47,* 839–853.

McCammon, S.L., & Allison E.J., Jr. (1995). Debriefing and treating emergency workers. In C. Figley (Ed.), *Compassion fatigue: Coping with secondary traumatic stress disorder in those who treat the traumatized* (pp. 115–130). New York: Brunner/Mazel.

McCann, I.L., Sakheim, D.K., & Abrahamson, D.J. (1988). Trauma and victimization: A model of psychological adaptation. *The Counseling Psychologist, 16,* 531–595.

Mounoud, P. (1976). The development of systems of representation and treatment in the child. In B. Inhelder and H. Chipman (Eds.), *Piaget and his school* (pp. 166–185). New York: Springer-Verlag.

Moyer, M.A. (1988). Achieving successful chemical dependency recovery in veteran survivors of traumatic stress. *Alcoholism Treatment Quarterly, 4*(4), 19–34.

Munroe, J.F., Shay, J., Fisher, L., Makary, C., Rapperport, K., & Zimering, R. (1995). Preventing compassion fatigue: A team treatment model. In C. Figley (Ed.), *Compassion fatigue: Coping with secondary traumatic stress disorder in those who treat the traumatized* (pp. 209–232). New York: Brunner/Mazel.

Orzek, A.M. (1983). Sexual assault: The female victim, her male partner and their relationship. *The Personnel and Guidance Journal, 62,* 143–146.

Pavalko, E.K., & Elder, G.H. (1990). World War II and divorce: A life-course perspective. *American Journal of Sociology, 95,* 1213–1234.

Pearlman, L.A., & Saakvitne, K.W. (1995). Treating therapists with vicarious traumatization and secondary traumatic stress disorders. In C. Figley (Ed.), *Compassion fatigue: Coping with secondary traumatic stress disorder in those who treat the traumatized* (pp. 150–177). New York: Brunner/Mazel.

Piaget, J. (1976). Biology and cognition. In B. Inheld and H. Chipman (Eds.). *Piaget and His School* (pp. 48–62). New York: Springer-Verlag.

Piaget, J., & Inhelder, B. (1969). *The psychology of the child.* New York: Basic Books.

Remer, P. (1984). *Stages in coping with rape.* Unpublished manuscript. Lexington: University of Kentucky.

Remer, R. (1990). *Secondary victim/Secondary survivor.* Unpublished manuscript. Lexington: University of Kentucky.

Remer, R., & Elliott, J.E. (1988a). Characteristics of secondary victims of sexual assault. *International Journal of Family Psychiatry, 9,* 373–387.

Remer, R., & Elliott, J.E. (1988b). Management of secondary victims of sexual assault. *International Journal of Family Psychiatry, 9,* 389–401.

Remer, R., & Ferguson, R.A. (1992a). *Counseling male partners of sexual assault victims: Producing secondary survivors.* Unpublished manuscript. Lexington: University of Kentucky.

Remer, R., & Ferguson, R.A. (1992b). *Becoming a secondary survivor of sexual assault.* Unpublished manuscript. Lexington: University of Kentucky.

Remer, R., & Ferguson, R.A. (1995). Becoming a secondary survivor of sexual assault. *Journal of Counseling and Development, 7,* 407–414.

Rodkin, L.I., Hunt, E.J., & Cowan, S.D. (1982). A men's support group for significant others of rape victims. *Journal of Marital and Family Therapy, 8,* 91–97.

Rosenheck, R., & Thomson, J. (1986). "Detoxification" of Vietnam war trauma: A combined family-individual approach. *Family Process, 25,* 559–570.

Scurfield, R. (1985). Post-trauma stress assessment and treatment: Overview and formulations. In C.R. Figley (Ed.), *Trauma and its wake: The study and treatment of post traumatic stress disorder* (pp. 219–255). New York: Brunner/ Mazel.

Smith-Schubert, S.C. (1985). The relationship of sex role orientation to anxiety, depression and marital adjustment among women who are wives or partners of Vietnam veterans identified as suffering delayed stress. *Dissertation Abstracts International, 46*(1-B), 315.

Solomon, Z. (1988). The effect of combat-related posttraumatic stress disorder on the family. *Psychiatry, 51,* 323–329.

Solomon, Z., Waysman, M., & Mikulincer, M. (1990). Family functioning, perceived societal support, and combat-related psychopathology: The moderating role of loneliness. *Journal of Social and Clinical Psychology, 9,* 456–472.

Steinberg, A. (1997). Understanding the secondary traumatic stress of children. In C. Figley (Ed.), *Burnout in families: The systemic costs of caring.* Boca Raton, FL: St. Lucie Press.

Sutherland, S., & Sherl, D.J. (1970). Patterns of response among victims of rape. *American Journal of Orthopsychiatry, 10,* 503–511.

Valent, P. (1995). Survival strategies: A framework for understanding secondary traumatic stress and coping in helpers. In C. Figley (Ed.), *Compassion fatigue: Coping with secondary traumatic stress disorder in those who treat the traumatized* (pp. 21–50). New York: Brunner/Mazel.

Whetsell, M.S. (1990). *The relationship of abuse factors and revictimization to the long-term effects of childhood sexual abuse in women.* Unpublished doctoral dissertation. Lexington: University of Kentucky.

Williams, M.B. (1997). Treating STSD in children. In C. Figley (Ed.), *Burnout in families: The systemic costs of caring.* Boca Raton, FL: St. Lucie Press.

Worell, J., & Remer, P. (1992). *Feminist perspectives in therapy: An empowerment model for women.* New York: John Wiley & Sons.

Yassen, J. (1995). Preventing secondary traumatic stress disorder. In C. Figley (Ed.), *Compassion fatigue: Coping with secondary traumatic stress disorder in those who treat the traumatized* (pp. 175–208). New York: Brunner/Mazel.

TREATING BURNOUT IN FAMILIES FOLLOWING CHILDHOOD TRAUMA

7

Michael F. Barnes, Ph.D.

INTRODUCTION

Bob is a 16-year-old male who had recently been admitted to a residential treatment facility due to severe emotional and behavioral problems. He entered this program with a long history of explosive, destructive, and aggressive outbursts of rage. Prior inpatient and outpatient treatment apparently had little impact on his patterns of destructive behaviors.

At our first meeting, it became evident that Bob's mother was very involved in his unsuccessful attempts at behavior change. Regardless of the questions asked, her discussion appeared to return to two primary themes. The first concerned how out of control and unpredictable her son's behavior had been. The second concerned how difficult it had been for her to fail in her attempts to control his destructive behaviors. She shared how confused and uncertain she felt when she searched for reasons for his behavior. She could identify no incidents of abuse or neglect, no early developmental crisis, or any subsequent medical illnesses.

When asked to talk about her other children, she stated that there was only one other child. She told of a 21-year-old son who also had a history of severe emotional and behavioral difficulties. After a brief

1-57444-047-0/98/$0.00+$.50

© 1998 by CRC Press LLC

171

pause in our discussion, this therapist asked again if there were any other children. Bob's mother hesitantly shared that she had one other son who was now deceased. He was one year younger than the oldest son and five years older than Bob. At the age of 15, he was struck by an automobile and sustained near-fatal injuries. She shared how she and the boys had to pull together to assist him through a long and difficult rehabilitation program. Fortunately, he recovered from his injuries and resumed the life of a normal teenager. Tragically, one year later, he was again struck by an automobile and died from his injuries.

When asked how her two surviving sons reacted to the death of their brother, she said that she did not know. She stated that they had never talked about it. She shared that she was so devastated by the death of her son that it was all she could do to keep her own life from falling apart. As time passed, there were so many emerging behavioral problems that she did not have time to delve into the boys' experiences of their brother's death.

As I wrote in Chapter 4 in this text, the incidence of traumatic injuries and death of children and adolescents in our society is staggering. Even in the most conscientious families, unexpected accidents and unthinkable acts of violence occur. Figley (1989) believes that most families find ways to positively support one another through their post-trauma responses. While all family members experience some type of post-trauma reaction, it is the social support between family members that prevents the formation of post-traumatic stress disorder (PTSD) and secondary traumatic stress disorder symptoms and any ongoing disruptions in the family structure and organization.

Unfortunately, many families, like the one discussed above, have difficulty supporting one another and struggle to identify satisfactory solutions for resolving a post-trauma crisis. In these cases, the unresolved crisis may result in a secondary traumatic stress response by the victim's family members (Barnes, 1995; Figley, 1995) as well as a disruption of the family system's structural and interactional functioning (Applebaum & Burns, 1991; Barnes, 1995; Madan-Swain, Sexson, Brown & Ragab, 1993; Rosenthal & Young, 1988; Waaland & Kreutzer, 1988; Zarski, DePompei & Zook, 1988).

It is also unfortunate that many of these traumatized families may not receive the needed therapeutic assistance for weeks, months, or even years following the traumatic event. There appear to be several reasons for this failure to treat traumatized families. One reason may be that certain types of traumatic events do not provide the family with an immediate opportunity to address the traumatic event. Barnes (1995) proposes that many families that experience the physical traumatization of a child may not receive therapeutic assistance because many hospitals do not provide services to the family during the child's hospitalization or following the child's discharge from the hospital setting. Also, many hospitals are very patient-focused and often fail to consider the secondary and systemic trauma experienced by the family members. This trauma impacts the overall well-being of the patient as well as the family.

A second reason may be that families that experience a traumatic event tend to develop covert and overt rules of silence following the traumatic event (Brende & Goldsmith, 1991), which prevents family members from trusting others to understand their pain. Some families enter a cycle of denial of painful feelings and build barriers between themselves and family members or the community. These barriers prohibit open communication. These feelings of alienation are often accompanied by a growing sense of shame and lower self-esteem associated with the feeling that they were unable to maintain the safety of their family member (Brende & Goldsmith, 1991).

A final reason may be that when traumatized families do seek therapeutic intervention, they often do so by "presenting a problem different than the traumatic event" (Figley, 1989, p. 43). Often these families will seek assistance for behavioral problems being exhibited by one or more of the children or for the relationship difficulties being experienced by the parents of the traumatized child. Until the therapist is able to identify the family history of unresolved trauma, the focus on the presenting problem may serve to camouflage the roots of the clinical issues and may provide fertile ground for therapy to become "stagnant" at some point later in the therapeutic process. It is critical that all therapists who work with trauma victims and their families understand the parallel processes of individual and systemic stress reactions that may occur and remain present for years following a traumatic event (Barnes, 1995).

This chapter begins with a discussion concerning some theoretical and epistemological issues associated with the use of family therapy for the treatment of traumatic stress issues. This is followed by a review of two models of family therapy that can assist the traumatized family to resolve the individual issues associated with both primary and secondary traumatic stress reactions. It is proposed that effective treatment begins with the two models reviewed. First, Structural Family Therapy

(Minuchin, 1974; Minuchin & Fishman, 1981) is utilized to address the family's structural reorganization associated with childhood traumatization. Secondly, Figley's Empowerment Model (Figley, 1989) is utilized to address primary and secondary trauma symptoms through the investigation of family members' subjective trauma experiences, which will ultimately lead to the development of a family healing theory.

FAMILY THERAPY AND THE TRAUMATIZED FAMILY

Traditional traumatology literature has focused on an individual's reactive symptoms development and the effectiveness of individually focused treatment models. At the same time, traditional family therapy practice models have focused on family interactional patterns and structural organization. Family therapists have traditionally avoided focusing on the symptoms associated with the "identified patient." The acceptance of secondary traumatization in the DSM-IV (APA, 1994) has challenged scholars and clinicians to reconceptualize PTSD treatment issues. It would appear that we can no longer look at the primary trauma victim as the root of family system dysfunction without also investigating the effect that the secondary traumatization of family members has had on the functioning of the family system.

This broadening of the trauma experience to include the secondary traumatization of family members is significant in that it moves the treatment of trauma from the individual to the family system context (Figley, 1989). This shift is also significant because it challenges the family therapist to move beyond the systemic concept of circular causality, to acknowledge that traumatic events can impact all individuals within a family system. These external events are experienced by individual family members and serve to influence individual and family world views associated with the traumatic event and often result in changes in the family organizational structure (Rosenthal & Young, 1988; Waaland & Kreutzer, 1988; Zarski, DePompei & Zook, 1988).

This movement from the individual to the system focus in treatment for traumatized families has not been as easily accepted as one might expect. Brooks (1991) states that while the classic struggle of family therapy since the 1950s has been to defocus attention from the "pathological identified patient" to the larger family system, much of the literature concerning family treatment for PTSD has continued to focus on the primary victim as the identified patient. Brooks (1991) suggests that a systemic focus can be maintained that will address the interactional patterns of the traumatized family while also acknowledging the extraordinary experiences of the primary trauma victim. From the standpoint of secondary traumatization, the family members' extraordinary experiences must also be acknowledged.

Some family therapists may question whether epistemological coherence can be maintained by using a treatment model that appears to be built upon a linear, cause-and-effect frame of reference. Wynne, Shields, and Sirkin (1992) contend that "illness, as traditionally understood in all cultures, is a relational, transactional concept that is highly congruent with core principles of present-day family theories" (p. 3). Illness can be conceptualized as a narrative or story about the subjective experiences and interactional behaviors associated with illness and disease within the family system. Wynne et al. (1992) propose that the concept of illness is individually and systemically constructed. It is the family's perception or world view associated with the illness that will dictate the interactional patterns associated with it.

These concerns are very important when dealing with the family of a traumatized child. Acknowledgment of each family member's painful experiences associated with the traumatic event must be made, while both supporting the family members and working on system interactional patterns.

COGNITIVE SCHEMAS, WORLD VIEW, AND FAMILY STRUCTURE

Alterations in cognitive schemas are clearly symptoms associated with individual PTSD and the focus of several effective individual treatment models (Bowen & Lambert, 1986; Janoff-Bulman, 1992; McCann & Pearlman, 1990; Scott & Stradling, 1992). Barnes (1995) and Figley (1995) propose that the family members of traumatized individuals experience their own secondary traumatization which, like PTSD, would include alterations in cognitive schemas. One can assume that the unique cognitive schemas associated with the traumatic event will be experienced by all family members and these will result in alterations in the family organization and structure. Minuchin and Fishman (1991) indicate that there is a clear relationship between alterations in family world view and alterations in family organization and structure. They propose that "any change in the family structure will change the family's world view, and any change in the world view will be followed by change in the family structure" (p. 207). A traumatic event impacts the family on both levels. Effective therapy utilizes interventions that will also enable the family to deal with issues of world view and family organization.

TREATING THE TRAUMATIZED FAMILY

McCann and Pearlman (1990) liken the therapy process to the "process of enlightenment" (p. 168). They propose that individuals should be encouraged to explore their disturbed schemas, to understand that altered schemas may be associated with increased difficulty in completing familiar tasks such as interpersonal interactions, and that altered schemas may be exhibited through changes in behavior or increased affect. For the family of a traumatized child, each of the above-stated points applies to the individual family members' unique trauma experience, as well as the family reorganization that is associated with the traumatic event. In the model that is proposed in the remaining pages of this chapter, a framework of Structural Family Therapy (Minuchin, 1974; Minuchin & Fishman, 1981) is utilized in the initial phases of treatment. This framework is utilized throughout the process of joining with the family, assessing the structural changes, and altered schemas associated with the trauma. Structural interventions are utilized to create a sense of order, safety, and control in the therapeutic setting, so that the family is ultimately prepared to address the specific traumatic event and its overall effect on the family.

Once the family trauma has been identified and each family member has accepted that it is at the root of their current emotional and behavioral difficulties, Figley's (1989) Empowerment Model is utilized to assist them in "making peace with the past." The Empowerment Model is built upon a complex foundation of crisis intervention theory, cognitive and behavioral psychology, and systems theory. It is a model that is designed to assist the family members in utilizing their natural strengths and coping abilities to resolve the painful memories and altered perceptions that are a result of the traumatic experience.

Joining with the Family

The most critical groundwork for intervention is the process of joining with the family. Colapinto (1991) refers to joining as the attention to simple "rules of etiquette, such as making friendly contact with all family members, confirmation of family members' expressions of concern, sadness, anger, fear, even rejection of therapy and maintenance of the rules that govern distance and hierarchies within the family system" (p. 437). When one considers the altered world views, concerns about safety and trust, and closing of system boundaries that occur following a traumatic event, joining with a traumatized family must be approached patiently. Care must be taken not to retraumatize the family by pushing too quickly to investigate the traumatic event. It is very important to let "the family know that the therapist understands them and is working with and for them. Only under this protection can the family have the security to explore alternatives, try the unusual, and change" (Minuchin & Fishman, 1981, pp. 31–32).

It is during this joining phase that the therapist must be clear in his or her understanding of the cause of these individual and family disturbances and articulate these beliefs to the family. Wynne et al. (1992) warn against the use of the traditional conception of "circular causality" when assessing the cause for illness, including illness associated with traumatic events. They cite two primary conceptual difficulties with family systems thinking for trauma therapy. The first is that the physical, sexual, or emotional abuse of a family member by another family member or outside individual allows for the identification of a responsible party or perpetrator. To place the responsibility anywhere other than on the perpetrator is "unfair and therapeutically inappropriate" (Wynne et al., 1992, p. 14). The second concern is that family members who seek professional assistance for a traumatized individual will experience blame if the therapist quickly turns his or her primary attention to family relationships rather than addressing the relevant concerns of the family.

On a personal note, after our son was nearly killed by an automobile several years ago, my wife and I spoke with a therapist about the traumatic experience. Following our initial session, we were amazed at how different our memories of the traumatic event and subsequent rehabilitation processes were. We were also amazed to look back and identify how conflicted our marital relationship and parenting practices had become. It became clear that we had greatly altered our subsystem boundaries by placing our son between us through a process of triangulation, which in turn influenced our communication patterns and decision-making processes. We were able to agree that it was the therapist's skill in joining with us that enabled us to experience the safety needed to talk about these painful issues. The therapist's active listening, normalizing, clarifying, and reframing of the trauma experience as being the result of a real and tragic event enhanced the joining process and reduced the chance of retraumatization.

Structural Paradigm for Working with World View

Minuchin and Fishman (1981) propose that there are four levels of communication/interaction between the therapist and the family that enable both to gain a better understanding of the individual and systemic world views that are held by the family. Therapeutic interaction at each level provides the therapist with different kinds of opportunities for understanding the family's world view associated with the presenting problem and to "intervene on" the interactional patterns that serve to maintain the primary, secondary, and systemic stress symptoms. Cognizance of these various levels of interaction is significant for the therapist who is attempting to assist families in integrating multiple independent world views into a new family world view or healing theory. These concepts are useful throughout the course of the therapeutic relationship with the family and are as important in dealing with structural reorganization as they are in healing the traumatic wounds.

The first level is the family's language and its influence on how the family is able to understand the traumatic event and its impact on their lives. The therapist must take care to note family language and investigate the meaning that individuals give to their descriptions of reality. This is consistent with the constructivist epistemology and allows the therapist to "ask questions which open the conversation to the elaboration of new meanings and communicative connections" (Goolishian & Winderman, 1988, p. 139).

The second level is the explanatory schemas, which include family "myths and history that organize both present and future" (Minuchin & Fishman, 1981, p. 211). Working with family myths allows valuable opportunities for evaluating the family's pre- and post-trauma functioning and for getting a glimpse of how the family believes life is supposed to be. This then becomes fertile ground for metaphors, reframes, and enactments geared toward changing communication patterns, hierarchical structures, and boundaries and ultimately individual world view. A respect for family myths and history will be very valuable later in the therapeutic process as the therapist assists the family in understanding the impact of the traumatic event on their belief systems, emotional experience, and interactional patterns. Simply asking questions regarding differences concerning past and present perceptions about the traumatized individual and the traumatizing event can provide the family with the opportunity to consider the traumatic material in unique ways, which produces previously unavailable insights and solutions to their current family problems.

The third level is that of explicit theory. At this level, the therapist assumes the role of expert. This role is especially helpful in working with the traumatized family members early in therapy as they thirst for information about normative responses to traumatic events. It also allows the therapist to begin noting observed examples of family strengths and competencies from the perspective of the expert who can see behavior patterns when clients cannot. Figley (1989) believes that the establishment of the therapist as a competent expert who has vast knowledge and experience in treating similar difficult cases is important in building rapport and enables the family members to feel safe enough to speak openly about the traumatic event.

The final level of intervention is through the utilization of the symbolic universe, where the therapist "presents interventions as if supported by an institution or consensus larger than the family" (Minuchin & Fishman, 1981, p. 215). The object is to utilize societal or universal truths as a means of reframing family and individual realities. In this case, the use of religious metaphors is often effective to reframe family beliefs concerning self or other blame and negative feelings concerning a lack of personal control over the situation. Clients with traumatized children often report that they are dealing with an uncertain future, possible lost dreams, and innumerable "what ifs!"

Structural Interventions

While McCann and Pearlman (1990) propose that clients should be gently encouraged to explore their disturbed schemas, Structural Family Therapy is often associated with confrontation and crisis induction rather than gentle encouragement, safety, and security. Colapinto (1991) asserts that the "structural approach to changing the family relies on the challenge to current patterns of transaction," but also warns that "challenge does not necessarily connote a harsh confrontation" (p. 438). Also, crisis induction does not always need to be completed with harsh, high-intensity interventions. Minuchin and Fishman (1981) state that "sometimes simple communications are simple enough" (p. 117). With families of traumatized children, crisis induction is an effective tool for altering transactional patterns, but the therapist must remain aware of the opportunity for retraumatization if rapport has not yet been developed and the family is not yet committed to the therapeutic process.

Minuchin and Fishman (1981) discuss the use of structural interventions to challenge the world view and constructed realities of client systems. Structural interventions such as enactment, unbalancing, crisis induction, and blocking are valuable tools in allowing family members to experience the emotions and interactional patterns associated with the presenting problem in a new and unique way. It is hypothesized that this new way of experiencing will lead to alternative understandings about the problem and the development of new and unique solutions.

Figley's Empowerment Model

Once the family members have come to accept that the traumatic event has resulted in emotional and behavioral changes that influence the way they interact as a family, the focus of the therapy can move to resolving the trauma. Again, this issue is best dealt with following the structural interventions that have served to create a family environment that is experienced as safe enough to talk about the painful memories, beliefs, and emotions associated with the traumatic event. To reiterate a point made in Chapter 4 in this text, issues may cover more than just the traumatic event. The family members may have to share their resentments at how much time parents spend away from the family, spouses may have to tell their partners how angry they are that they had to deal with so much of the trauma alone, children may have to share resentment at having to take over parental responsibility, or one spouse may have to share how much it hurt to not be a part of an enmeshed relationship between the traumatized child and the other parent. In order to truly resolve the trauma and remove the primary, secondary, and systemic symptoms that are associated with it, each family member will need to tell his or her story. They must be able to do this without interruption and without the need to defend their position.

Figley's (1989) Empowerment Model is a five-stage model that is designed to allow family members to reexperience the traumatic event, to identify and contemplate their emotional and cognitive responses to the event, and to then work together to make sense of the incident and its impact on them as a family. The initial step of this model calls for the therapist to work with the family to build a commitment to the therapeutic objectives. Within the model that has been put forth in this chapter, it would be assumed that the therapeutic relationship has already been established through the assessment and structural phases. Like Minuchin and Fishman (1981), Figley believes that it is important for the therapist to be seen as an expert who is competent in working with these types of difficult trauma cases. Ultimately it is critical to establish in this phase the family's ability to articulate the major sources of stress endured by the family and to identify specific treatment objectives.

The second stage of the model is a time for framing the problem. Figley (1989) states that "memory management is the key ingredient in recovery from post-traumatic stress disorder" (p. 78). Therefore, it is the task of the therapist to assist the family in recalling important bits of information about the traumatic event and to then "help them manage, restructure, and reframe this information" (Figley, 1989, p. 78).

The first task of this second stage is to allow each member of the family to tell his or her whole story concerning the traumatic event. These stories must be uninterrupted by other family members and not edited by the storyteller. This is a time to talk about personal perceptions associated with the crisis and the negative disruptions that have been experienced. Figley (1989) states that this is a time for promoting new rules of communication, understanding, and acceptance; identification of trauma-related consequences; an opportunity for social support; and a shift in attention from the primary victim/patient to the family. The goal of this stage of therapy is to "begin to identify the building blocks for a healing theory, a statement of what, how, and why this terrible thing happened" (Figley, 1989, p. 86). It must be noted that this may be a difficult stage for the family members. As each shares his or her story, it may be received by the other family members as attacking, blaming, and painful. Even if family members do not agree with the speaker's experience of the traumatizing event, the therapist must not allow the others to interrupt. It is important for the family members to understand that all aspects of the family experience of the trauma must be placed on the table, where they can be dealt with in an open and honest fashion.

The major task of the third stage is to assist the family in reframing the problem. In this stage, the therapist assists the family members in reaching some consensus about their views of the traumatic experience and in beginning to identify new frames through which the family can begin to conceptualize new, more manageable and functional, coping behaviors. Once the family members can begin to perceive the trauma differently, they can begin to identify alternative coping strategies. Families can begin to see the challenge that has been presented to them through this terrible circumstance.

The fourth stage of the model is the establishment of individual family-member healing theories, which will ultimately be utilized in the development of a family healing theory. It appears that this healing theory emerges as the family members continue the process of open communication about the event, while simultaneously experiencing support from the other members of the family. Ultimately, it is in this stage that the family members are assisted in the process of stating their understanding of the new meaning that the event has begun to have for them. The individual sharing becomes a therapeutic conversation, with an ongoing process culminating in a co-created family healing theory. Figley (1989) proposes that many highly functioning families will be able to develop this healing theory naturally in time after the experience of a trauma.

Once the family is able to articulate its mutually agreed upon healing theory, they are ready to begin the process of closure. During this stage, the therapist and family should review and discuss the treatment goals that have been successfully completed, including the treatment goals that were established early in the therapy, associated with structural and interactional changes that have enabled the family to begin the process of talking about this painful event. The therapist and family should also identify family social-support systems and begin to make suggestions about new rules and skills of family communication that may assist them in continuing on their path to recovery.

CONCLUSION

I will never forget the sick feeling in my stomach and the immediate feeling of terror as the policeman informed me that my son had been hit by a car. My wife will never forget watching him run across the street and be hit by that car. She will never forget those moments immediately following the accident in which she said that she felt nothing, but could only wonder if I would stay in school now that Patrick was dead.

Although the victim was the same five-year-old boy, we had two very different experiences of the traumatic event. It was sudden, unexpected, and in the hours, days, weeks, and months following the accident impacted every aspect of our lives and our relationships. Since that time, I have studied the impact of trauma on the family and have worked with many traumatized families. I continue to be amazed by the resiliency of these families and have come to understand what I have heard Dr. Figley say many times in the past, that the response to trauma "is a very normal response to a very abnormal circumstance."

For the therapist who works with traumatized families, it is critical to understand the family's experience of the traumatic event and the struggle of each family member to understand and cope with the multiple stressors that are now impacting their daily thoughts, feelings, and relationships. Respect must be shown for the families presenting problems, whether they are initially concerned with the acting out of a sibling, mother's depression, or the traumatic event itself. As the program director of a residential treatment facility for adolescent boys, I find that most families are like Bob's (discussed at the beginning of this chapter), in that they are very concerned about their children and want them to receive the best possible treatment. I also find that although most of these families have been through multiple treatment resources which have addressed the traumatic events experienced by the troubled youth, most have not addressed the cognitive and emotional impact of these traumatizing events on the family as a unit. I find that in addressing these issues with families, care must be taken not to retraumatize the family by too quickly moving the focus to systemic functioning as the cause of the boy's ongoing difficulties. A process of normalizing the family's response to the catastrophic life event is important in order for the family to feel that they are being heard.

What is especially positive about the use of these two models of family therapy is that they have been found to be effective in assisting families to identify and change the response patterns that have commonly been attributed to the families of traumatized or ill children. The Structural Family Therapy model allows the family to begin the process of reorganization that will create the safety and trust needed to begin working on the painful trauma memories. Figley's model encourages family members to experience and discuss their painful affect, to acknowledge and share their perceptions of the event and the consequences that they have experienced. It urges families to break the rules of silence and resume the process of family social support. It also addresses the significant issue of family perception of stressors, allowing family members to create new perceptions and new solutions to their problems.

REFERENCES

American Psychiatric Association (1994). *Diagnostic and statistical manual of mental disorders* (4th ed.). Washington, DC: American Psychiatric Association.

Applebaum, D.R., & Burns, G.L. (1991). Unexpected childhood death: Posttraumatic stress disorder in surviving sibling and parents. *Journal of Clinical Child Psychology, 20*(2), 114–120.

Barnes, M.F. (1995). *The impact of the physical traumatization and critical care hospitalization of children, on the functioning of the injured child's family system: A delphi study.* Unpublished doctoral dissertation. Tallahassee: Florida State University.

Bowen, G.R., & Lambert, J.A. (1986). Systematic desensitization therapy with post-traumatic stress disorder cases. In C.R. Figley (Ed.), *Trauma and its wake, Volume II: Traumatic stress theory, research and intervention* (pp. 280–291). New York: Brunner/Mazel.

Brende, J.O., & Goldsmith, R. (1991). Post-traumatic stress disorder in families. *Journal of Contemporary Psychotherapy, 21*(2), 115–124.

Brooks, G.R. (1991). Therapy pitfalls with Vietnam veteran families: linearity, contextual naiveté, and gender role blindness. *Journal of Family Psychology, 4*(4), 446–461.

Colapinto, J. (1991). Structural Family Therapy. In A.S. Gurman and D.P. Kniskern (Eds.), *Handbook of family therapy* (revised) (pp. 417–443). New York: Brunner/Mazel.

Figley, C.R. (1989). *Helping traumatized families.* San Francisco: Jossey-Bass.

Figley, C.R. (1995). Compassion fatigue as secondary traumatic stress disorder: An overview. In C.R. Figley (Ed.), *Compassion fatigue: Secondary traumatic stress disorder in treating the traumatized.* New York: Brunner/Mazel.

Goolishian, H.A., & Winderman, L. (1988). Constructivism, autopoiesis and problem determined systems. *The Irish Journal of Psychology, 9*(1), 130–143.

Janoff-Bulman, R. (1992). *Shattered assumptions: Towards a new psychology of trauma.* New York: The Free Press.

Madan-Swain, A., Sexson, S.B., Brown, R.T., & Ragab, A. (1993). Family adaptation and coping among siblings of cancer patients, their brothers and sisters, and nonclinical controls. *The American Journal of Family Therapy, 21*(1), 60–71.

McCann, I.L., & Pearlman, L.A. (1990). *Psychological trauma and the adult survivor: Theory, therapy, and transformation.* New York: Brunner/Mazel.

Minuchin, S. (1974). *Families and family therapy.* Cambridge, MA: Harvard University Press.

Minuchin, S., & Fishman, H.C. (1981). *Family therapy techniques.* Cambridge, MA: Harvard University Press.

Rosenthal, M., & Young, T. (1988). Effective family intervention after traumatic brain injury: Theory and practice. *Journal of Head Trauma Rehabilitation, 3*(4), 42–50.

Scott, M.J., & Stradling, S.G. (1992). *Counseling for post-traumatic stress disorder.* Newberry Park, CA: Sage.

Waaland, P.K., & Kreutzer, J.S. (1988). Family response to childhood traumatic brain injury. *Journal of Head Trauma Rehabilitation, 3*(4), 51–63.

Wynne, L.C., Shields, C.G., & Sirkin, M.I. (1992). Illness, family theory and family therapy. I: Conceptual issues. *Family Process, 31*(3), 3–18.

Zarski, J.J., DePompei, R., & Zook, A. (1988). Traumatic head injury: Dimensions of family responsivity. *Journal of Head Trauma Rehabilitation, 3*(4), 31–41.

TREATING TRAUMATIZED FAMILIES

8

Donald R. Catherall, Ph.D.

INTRODUCTION

It is increasingly clear that relating to a trauma survivor can produce symptoms of traumatic stress in professionals who work closely with survivors (Figley, 1995). The same is obviously true for family members; the difference is that family members cannot escape to the sanctuary of their homes while they reconstitute for another day's stressful contact. Because they either live with or are highly accessible to the survivor, and because they have the most intimate dealings with the survivor, family members are exposed at a level that exceeds that of everyone else in the survivor's life. Fortunately, those same family members tend to care more than others involved with the survivor and are thus motivated to tolerate a great deal of stress. However, like anyone else, the more they are exposed, the greater the likelihood they will be affected. Moreover, because they are a family system, they are not only individually affected but are also affected as a group. The more some members of the family are secondarily traumatized, the greater the likelihood that the entire environment of the family will suffer. When the family can be characterized as traumatized, then the family environment can be characterized as burned out.

The basic model for treating a traumatized family is based upon the model of recovery that is generally accepted for traumatized individuals. A central tenet of the traumatization model is that recovery is a natural

1-57444-047-0/98/$0.00+$.50

process that occurs when people have an interpersonal environment in which they can safely discuss and examine their experience on both cognitive and emotional levels. The recovery process includes the expression of significant affects, particularly grief, and usually leads to the acquisition of a new cognitive perspective on the traumatic experience (Figley, 1989). Often, the individual's entire world view shifts during the recovery process. The primary job of the therapist is to facilitate the establishment and maintenance of a safe recovery environment.

In this chapter, the traumatization model is amended in two ways. First, the focus is on the family rather than the individual. Second, the concept of recovery is used in regard to the burnout environment itself, as distinguished from recovery from traumatization per se. Herman (1992) characterizes the recovery process of traumatized individuals in stages, beginning with a stage of establishing safety, moving through a stage of mourning and memory processing, and culminating in a stage of reconnecting. Although this model describes the general process of change seen in some families, it does not reflect the process of recovery from a burned-out environment so much as recovery from traumatization. As with recovery from traumatization, a family's recovery from a burned-out family environment begins with the establishment of greater safety and moves toward greater connectedness (Herman's first and third stages). However, many family members do not have a clearly defined middle stage in which they will mourn and do memory work. Indeed, some family members may have no memories or limited knowledge of the trauma or may not have any experience of a non-burned-out family environment. More often, the middle stage of recovery from the burnout environment consists of identifying and changing dysfunctional mechanisms and patterns in the family. During that stage, the therapist is often required to challenge existing interaction patterns and unwritten rules that control family behavior. In order to have an environment in which dysfunctional mechanisms and patterns can be challenged, the therapist first must create a safe environment where family members learn to operate by different rules.

SECONDARY TRAUMATIZATION OF FAMILIES

In traumatized families, it is assumed that one or more members of the family were traumatized via exposure to a trauma (the primary stressor) and that the other members of the family have themselves either (1) been traumatized as a result of their exposure to the traumatized member(s) (the secondary stressor) or (2) been affected as a result of growing up in the burned-out environment that developed in the family subsequent to the traumatization. In some cases, the primary trauma may have happened to members of an earlier generation, and those family members may even be deceased. Yet the family can still be burned out and continuing to burn out new family members. For example, stories of the trauma of earlier generations may be passed along in the family. The stories themselves may be traumatizing, but even more important are the lessons gleaned from the stories. Through the medium of such stories, new family members are inculcated with the "family perception", the family's idiosyncratic view of the world (e.g., an unsafe place where strangers are not to be trusted).

TREATING THE WHOLE FAMILY SYSTEM

Previous chapters in this volume have focused on the treatment of various burned-out components of the family system (i.e., children, spouses, and parents). The goal of this chapter is to focus on the treatment of the traumatized family as a whole. Taking this point of view allows us to attend to aspects of the family environment that affect every member but are not easily attributed to any single member. These aspects are seldom well understood or easily identified by the family, yet they are implicit in the family's daily life and they are manifested in the family's communication patterns. These aspects reflect underlying attitudes and beliefs of individual family members, but they are sustained at a level of interactive reality that is superordinate to the conscious beliefs and attitudes of individual members. Consequently, it is very difficult to change these aspects of family life, as no individual seems to be responsible for them but everyone participates in maintaining them.

This chapter identifies those mechanisms that define and maintain the burnout environment, as well as the features of the desired recovery environment. The goal is to provide therapists with a model of an effective recovery environment and a lens that will aid them to quickly recognize the family's blocks against an effective recovery environment. The chapter is thus organized to provide a lens to help therapists see these vital mechanisms rather than as a how-to manual on changing those mechanisms. The focus is on the ultimate goals of intervening rather than on particular styles of intervening. Hence, this chapter will not focus on specific intervention techniques but instead will focus on those aspects of the family environment that must change in order to create a safe and effective recovery environment. Several examples will be given in order to provide a sense of how these mechanisms are manifested and what the change process looks like.

Description of the Burnout Environment

The environment of a traumatized family is ultimately sterile. Whether the family members are disengaged or engaged in conflict, are inexpressive or express affection, are depressed or lead busy productive lives, there is still something missing in the home environment. That something is the spontaneous, authentic, real presence of each family member. Each member is less than fully there. Significant aspects of each family member's full range of emotions, thoughts, and needs are missing. The result is that family members do not really feel connected with one another. They do not know each other in the complete manner that is possible for people whose lives are intimately connected.

A model that focuses on the importance of "connected" relationships has been developed by members of the Stone Center at Wellesley College (Jordan et al., 1991). This relational model of development is intended to capture the unique features of women's development (Jordan, 1989). The relational model of development recasts the role of the therapist in the therapy relationship—emphasizing the importance of mutuality in the therapist–client relationship (Stiver, 1991; Jordan, 1991b; Miller & Stiver, 1991). The model posits that (women's) development only occurs within a relationship; that is, growth occurs in connection. This process is seen as an ongoing need, not something that is accomplished once and forever. In order to develop fully, the person (woman) must be able to bring all of her or his experience into the connection. To the degree that significant aspects of an individual's experience are kept out of the connection, then the relationship will be superficial and the individual will not be able to grow adequately. In a traumatized family, significant aspects of every family member's experience are kept out of the connections.

There are several common features of the unconnected, traumatized family system. There is a general lack of authenticity; no member has the experience of feeling fully understood because no member reveals all of herself or himself to the others. Expressivity is constricted; some or many emotions are simply never expressed. For some families, this may mean that a few very vulnerable emotions stay underground. For others, it can mean that emotionality per se is not allowed and the atmosphere is consequently dry and unemotional. In either case, there is a lack of emotional accessibility in the parents (Stiver, 1990a).

Relationships in a disconnected family are not mutual or reciprocal (Jordan, 1991a). Instead, there is a tendency for family members to assume fixed roles, such as the many inflexible roles identified in alcoholic families. There is a lack of effective conflict resolution, that is, no process of resolving conflicts that respects the needs and feelings of all family members. Finally, though some of these families may be contained within a rigid boundary (against the outside world), there is a lack of feelings of true closeness within the family.

Stiver (1990b) discusses "strategies of disconnection" in dysfunctional, traumatized families, noting that family members learn ways of being together while simultaneously remaining disconnected. This allows family members to protect those vulnerable parts of themselves that they do not feel safe exposing, while still maintaining some kind of connection. These disconnection strategies can themselves become problems and often contribute to other forms of dysfunctional coping. Operating in disconnected relationships and employing dysfunctional coping strategies places the family at increased risk in any future encounters with traumatic stress.

Ineffective Coping Reactions

The burnout environment initially develops as a result of the family's failure to effectively recover from the traumatization of one or more members. The most common reason that the recovery process gets stymied is that the family lacks the kind of effective coping that enhances recovery. Figley and McCubbin (1983) note that the family both reacts to and produces stress, thus either undermining or contributing to the functioning of family members. They have identified several coping strategies that vary with the degree of a family's functionality vs. dysfunctionality (McCubbin & Figley, 1983). Dysfunctional strategies include *ineffective problem solving* (i.e., failing to effectively identify stressors and being blame-oriented rather than solution-oriented). They noted the importance of *communication problems*, such as indirect, closed communication and a lack of tolerance for idiosyncratic expressions and behavior. They also noted problems in the *family structure* (i.e., a lack of cohesion, rigidity of roles, and the tendency to view problems as centered in an individual rather than family-centered). Finally, they noted that dysfunctional families are less effective at utilizing resources and may resort to problem-producing strategies of violence and drug usage.

INTERVENING IN THE BURNOUT ENVIRONMENT

Families that rely upon dysfunctional coping strategies are handicapped in their ability to effectively engage in the work of recovery—in processing the event and mourning the many losses associated with it. The family's failure to process and mourn leads to three general areas of dysfunction: (1) the family's connections—a breakdown in the family's ability to care for its members, (2) the family's reality—the development of distortions in the family's consensual reality, and (3) the family's symptoms—the continuation of issues related to the actual trauma. Within each of the three areas are specific elements that serve to maintain the burnout environment. These elements and their associated mechanisms are the targets for therapeutic change. The overall level of connectedness between family members tends to improve as these areas of dysfunction improve.

There are other mechanisms that are common foci of family therapy with dysfunctional families and are frequently awry in the burnout environment, but they do not appear to play such a central role in defining the specific trauma-related nature of the environment. These mechanisms include boundary problems (Minuchin, 1982), lack of differentiation (Bowen, 1966), and the general systems notions of homeostasis and deviation-reducing and deviation-amplifying (feedback) mechanisms (Jackson, 1957; Maruyama, 1963). Family therapy of a traumatized family is likely to involve any of these, as well as other traditional foci of family therapy. However, for the purposes of this chapter, we will focus on those elements and mechanisms that seem to play a more central role in defining and maintaining the burnout environment in families affected by trauma.

Levels of Intervention

The first level of intervention is manifested in the structure of the therapeutic environment (i.e., the family is trained to communicate

more effectively and use functional coping strategies while in the presence of the therapist). This level of intervention is the same for all
families because the same rules of functional coping and effective
communication are pursued regardless of a family's specific problems.
Family therapists typically conduct their sessions according to functional
modes of communication and problem solving and challenge any dysfunctional coping patterns that they encounter.

The second level of intervention involves the therapist's focus on the
mechanisms that maintain the burnout environment. These mechanisms
are recurring patterns that both manifest and reinforce the beliefs,
attitudes, and behaviors that compose the burnout environment. Family
therapists have long focused on recurring patterns because of the role
they play in maintaining family problems (Feldman & Pinsof, 1982).
Family therapy generally involves confronting and changing these pat-
terns/mechanisms.

Targeted Areas of Change

The targeted elements and mechanisms are derived from: (1) the disrupted connections, (2) the distorted reality, and (3) the unresolved
trauma issues. Figure 8.1 shows the elements targeted for change and
the central effects of each of these problem areas. Within the area of
disrupted connections, the elements targeted for change are (a) the
emotional inaccessibility between family members, particularly the inaccessibility of the parents, and (b) the parentification of the children.
Within the area of the distorted family reality, the targeted elements are
(a) the distorted world view, (b) family myths about the event, and (c)
the dysfunctional rules that stem from the myths and world view.
Within the area of specific trauma-related symptoms/issues, the targeted
elements are (a) the reenactments and projections related to the trauma,
(b) the continuing concerns about safety, (c) the survivor missions
assumed by family members, and (d) the continued symptomatic behavior of affected family members.

The immediate goal of the therapy is to change those targeted
elements that are awry and that play a central role in maintaining the
burnout environment. As the burnout environment changes, the family
may then proceed to finish the interrupted processing and mourning of
the trauma, if it is still relevant to do so. For some families, the original
trauma may no longer be relevant (e.g., it happened to generations that
are now deceased). Other families may continue to need the therapist's

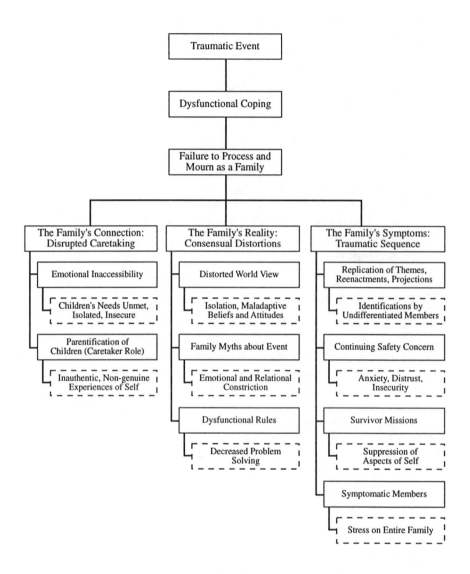

Figure 8.1   Affected Areas of Family Functioning which Require Intervention

help with the actual processing. In either case, the ultimate goal of the therapy is to achieve a level of connection that enables each family member to be fully genuine and present.

The following sections discuss the targeted mechanisms in greater depth in order to give therapists a clear grasp of what they are trying to change. Several examples will be presented to make the process more tangible.

The Family's Connectedness: Failures in Caretaking

One of the central elements that defines the traumatized family is the lack of connectedness among family members. This lack of connectedness in turn interferes with one of the defining aspects of family life— the capacity of family members to be emotionally attuned and responsive to one another. The lack of emotional attunement and responsiveness leads to failures in the family's ability to take care of its members.

Emotional Inaccessibility

One of the most common sequelae of traumatization is the development of alexithymia, a condition in which individuals are unable to effectively identify and express a wide range of emotions and often experience their emotions in the form of regressed somatic states (Krystal, 1988). The alexithymic nature of the traumatized family members and the many rules controlling the expression of emotions create an atmosphere of emotional constriction and emotional blindness that interferes with proper attunement between family members, particularly the attunement of parents to children. Due to their own emotional blocks, parents may misperceive their children's emotions. This can have a lasting effect because the child is learning to know his or her feelings. Donovan and McIntyre note how the nature and meaning of emotions are "negotiated" between mother and infant and how that process then bears upon the child's development:

> Infant discomfort due to hunger or pain, for example, can be mis-interpreted, misidentified and mislabeled by mother in terms of emotions or attitudes such as anger, hatred, or rejection. We see here the potential for the attribution of intent, which can become extremely confusing for the developing infant and child and significantly confuse the notion of agency (1990, p. 56).

When the therapist has access to the family, the therapist endeavors to: (1) help the parents identify what each child is feeling, (2) help the children identify what they are feeling, (3) help all family members express their feelings, and (4) coach the parents to respond to the children's feelings. In the case of a severely alexithymic family, the therapist usually has to be very active in identifying feelings for the family members, as they can be quite limited in their ability to recognize their own feeling states.

The therapist can quickly gain access to the feeling dimension with the family through the medium of the presenting problem. Using a problem-centered approach, the therapist explores how each family member views the problem, what each has done to try to solve the problem, and how each member feels about the problem (Catherall, 1988). If members question the relevance of exploring feelings about the problem, the therapist can talk about the role feelings play in problem solving. Pinsof explains the need for exploration of emotions in effective problem solving:

> Emotions facilitate action or behavior. Specifically, emotions either facilitate or inhibit effective problem solving. They also add genuineness, intensity, vitality, and spontaneity to problem solving. Without emotion, problem solving becomes an empty, primarily cognitive endeavor that is seldom integrated or enduring (1995, p. 174).

As the family's awareness of feelings increases, the therapist begins to probe family members' ability to read each others' feelings. This leads to increased communication between family members as the members learn to check out their perceptions and assumptions about each others' feelings. A related goal of the exploration of feelings and communication work is to increase the experience of empathy between family members, particularly the parents' ability to empathize with the children.

The Parentification of Children: Altering Family Roles

Many dysfunctional roles evolve in families that have constricted means of managing extreme emotions. In such families, the parents are usually unable to provide the full spectrum of parenting, leaving significant gaps in areas such as nurturance, modeling, limit setting, managing resources, and, perhaps most commonly, being emotionally accessible. If there are enough children, they tend to try to fulfill all the parenting gaps, but, of course, they pay a price for this premature development. Some children assume adult levels of responsibility by becoming some variant of a parentified child (i.e., emotional caretaker, surrogate spouse, breadwinner, homemaker, etc.) (Stiver, 1990a). Other children often adopt irresponsible roles that express the family's conflicts and draw attention to the denied feelings and needs (see "Replication of Trauma Themes", page 204).

The unfortunate outcome for so many children who fulfill these rigid roles is that the child's personality becomes confused with the family role. As adults, these individuals generally experience psychotherapy as liberating because it frees them up from a role that is no longer adaptive. In the best of outcomes, they regain the freedom to be authentic and to bring all parts of themselves into the connection with the other family members. If therapists have access to the family while the children are still young, the goal is to help the parents recover their ability to do their job and be emotionally accessible. If the therapy is being conducted with an individual who was parentified in childhood, then the goal is to help that person identify and pursue his or her own needs, set limits in relationships, and quit being an exclusive caretaker. Caretakers typically ignore their own needs in their rush to take care of others. If the therapy is being conducted with an individual who was the recipient of familial projections and was pulled into traumatic reenactments, then the goal is to help that person distinguish his or her true self from the negative role played in the family. Such individuals usually have problems with self-esteem and are very harsh with themselves.

Example

David H was one of four sons whose father died when David was nine years old. David was with his father when he died in an accident. Although the youngest child in the family, David was the most involved with his father in his routines of taking care of the property. After his father's death, David continued to perform his father's duties around the house. Soon, he began keeping an eye on his older brothers and took on parenting responsibilities regarding them. He did things like staying up late until they returned home at night, accompanying them to parties to see that they did not drink excessively, and chastising them if they created problems for the family. David's own needs became submerged beneath his constant vigil over the rest of the family. He regarded his mother as overwhelmed and consequently made no demands upon her.

As an adult, David became depressed after having an auto accident on the anniversary of his father's death. He had created a marital relationship in which he viewed his wife as fragile, took care of her, and "protected" her from his own needs and feelings. The result was that he felt just as alone and overwhelmed as he did as a nine-year-old. Further, he himself had come to view his personality as the same as his caretaker role. He didn't need anything from others and couldn't see how emotional support would make any difference. Psychotherapy helped David discover the many parts of himself that were hidden by his clinging to his father through living his father's role and responding to his mother's emotional inaccessibility by becoming the family caretaker himself.

The Family's Reality: Cognitive Distortions

Every distinct human system develops its own unique view of reality. That view may vary from the view maintained by surrounding systems to a greater or lesser degree, depending in part upon how open or closed the system is in respect to the reality orientation of the surrounding systems. For example, within American culture there are numerous subcultural groups, some of which are more closed to the values and mores of the Judeo-Christian culture that predominates in middle-class America. The result is that some of these closed systems are thus able to maintain views of reality that are distinctly non-mainstream (e.g., beliefs that subgroups are secretly ruling the world or that individuals can be controlled by people with supernatural powers).

Every family exists within some larger cultural group. When the family is closed, then the views of the surrounding culture have less influence on the family's personal view of reality and the reality orientations promoted within the family. The older members of the family play a key role in introducing the younger, less differentiated members to the family's view of reality. As in all groups, family members shape and mutually reinforce each others' views through agreement, challenge, skepticism, reward, punishment, and the like. The result of this process of convergence is a consensual view of reality that exists within every family. However, the more closed the family is, the less heterogeneous that consensual reality and the more likely it will diverge from the reality orientation of the surrounding culture.

The attitudes, beliefs, and reality attributions made by individuals exposed to trauma play a critical role in determining the meaning given to the trauma, just as their cultural heritage plays an important role in empowering their specific healing rituals (Wilson, 1989). Although the knowledge in this area is largely anecdotal and not yet based upon a body of scientific research, it appears likely that some events experienced as traumatic in one cultural setting may be experienced as non-traumatic in a different cultural setting. This is because the meaning attributed to events can vary according to one's view of reality. For example, in ancient Sparta teenage boys were frequently beaten by adults, usually their parents. The meaning given that experience in that warrior culture was that it helped the boys become stronger and able to endure pain. Hence, it is likely that being beaten was not experienced as traumatic as often in that cultural context as it would be in modern American culture, where it would be seen as a form of abuse.

Traumatized families tend to become closed and develop specific idiosyncratic interpretations of their world (their world view) that may be at considerable variance from the views of surrounding systems. Within their closed internal world, they have their own values, mores, customs, rituals, and ways of operating and behaving. Children growing up in one of these encapsulated family systems acquire the family's unique view of reality, which can cause dissonance when the child interacts with surrounding systems.

Distorted World View

A family that has been burned out for a period of time develops attitudes, beliefs, and an overall world view that, once established, interfere with the members' ability to fully engage in relationships and instead sustain the burnout environment. This consensually derived world view is shared by family members and is implicit in many different forms of family communication. The attitudes and beliefs that compose the dysfunctional world view primarily involve safety, the self, others, and the meaning of life.

Questions of safety focus on the conditions under which a member of this family can feel safe or should feel unsafe. The conditions of safety usually relate directly to the primary trauma and the family's attributions concerning its cause.

Attitudes and beliefs regarding the self focus on issues of identity, self-worth, and self-competence. Who are we? How do we have good feelings about ourselves? Must self-worth be earned? If so, how is it earned? What must one accomplish or endure in order to feel competent to deal with life?

Attitudes and beliefs regarding others focus on issues of trust, dependability, and human nature. Who can be trusted? Who is not trustworthy? How much should one trust others? What are the advantages and perils of trusting? To what degree can others be depended upon? When others let a person down, is it viewed as a minor aspect of human nature or is it a betrayal that cannot be forgiven? What is the basic view of human nature? Are people basically good? Are some evil? How does the family explain the existence of people like the perpetrators of the Holocaust?

Attitudes and beliefs regarding the meaning of life include values and priorities. What makes life meaningful? Is it necessary to have a mission or a sense of duty? Is grace gained through suffering or is life to be enjoyed to the fullest? How does one explain the occurrence of tragedy in people's lives? Who is more important—the individual, the family, or the community?

Figley has noted that individual recovery from traumatization is usually reflected in a shift of perspective regarding issues such as the individual's role in the primary trauma (Figley, 1988, 1989). In families, recovery from a burnout state is reflected in a shift of perspective in the family's beliefs and attitudes concerning safety, the self, others, and the meaning of life. The therapist facilitates this shift in the family's world view by (1) helping them see how these beliefs and attitudes developed as a result of the trauma, (2) helping them recognize when their behavior is reflecting the trauma-derived beliefs and attitudes, and (3) helping them use the safety of the therapeutic setting to explore alternative operational hypotheses about their world.

Family Myths

A major mechanism that defines and maintains the trauma-related themes in families is the family myth. Through the medium of family stories, newer family members (generally children, but also adults who join the family, usually through marriage) are introduced to the family's self-definition. The family stories teach these new members such central aspects of self-definition as who we are, how we behave, what we believe, and what the themes are that define our lives. The family myths are the lessons that are gleaned from the traumatic events captured in the family stories.

The family myth "evolves out of traumatic, life-threatening experiences which elicit shared decisions that have survival value at the time" (Kramer, 1985, p. 13). These decisions have short-term value but can interfere with family life if they become a long-term operating guideline. Jan Kramer gives an example of such a myth from her own family of origin:

> The myth—Mother is fragile: she may die if she does not get her way—evolved out of the traumatic, life threatening experiences the family shared around Mother's depression and hospitalization following my father's inaccessibility and the deaths of my paternal grandmother and baby sister. These traumas elicited a shared decision—Not to disagree with or question Mother—that had survival value at the time...As I did not question the myth, it continued to dominate my life, interfering in my interactions with my husband and children (pp. 187–188).

A helpful tactic in family therapy is to search out the significant family stories and give words to the myths that may have evolved out of the family traumas. When family members are able to observe the myths that have ruled their lives, they have more choice over the rules by which they will live. Family diagramming can be helpful in capturing this kind of information.

Family Rules

Unearthing family myths reveals some of the dysfunctional rules that guide family behavior. Family therapists have long focused on the unwritten rules that can be inferred by studying the family's behavior. The family myth captures those rules that developed as a direct consequence of the family's traumatic experience. The primary area in which maladaptive rules interfere with the appropriate processing of trauma is in the family's expression of emotion. However, in the burnout environment, many rules develop that maintain the environment.

In addition to defining what kinds of emotions can and cannot be expressed, family rules regulate behaviors that involve issues such as vulnerability (e.g., help seeking, apologizing, compromise), power, conflict, affection, and familial cohesion. Traumatized families frequently manifest dysfunctional rules in many of these areas through the use of family secrets (Stiver, 1990b). Secrets can control access between members, define inappropriate boundaries, uphold corrupt power structures, and interfere with cohesion.

Rules specifying the functioning of family members may be general to all family members or specific to individual members or subgroups. In the burnout environment, maladaptive general rules always exist and maladaptive rules applying to individuals and subgroups usually exist as well. For example, in the same family different rules may be directed toward: (1) different subgroups (e.g., men, parents, children), (2) different individuals/roles (e.g., mother, grandfather, etc.), or (3) everyone in the system. Thus, the rules of the family might include: men don't cry, mother is never taken seriously, and no one in the family reveals weakness. As with giving words to the myths, the therapist's overt identification of the rules provides family members an opportunity to choose the rules by which they will live.

The Family's Symptoms: Traumatic Sequelae

The third area in which the traumatized family carries on the effects of the trauma consists of the various traumatic feelings and symptoms. These range from the symptomatic behavior of traumatized members to excessive concerns about safety to the pursuit of trauma-related life goals. In these different ways, the original trauma continues to hold sway over the family's life.

Replication of Trauma Themes

One way in which elements of a trauma are passed on in a family is through the recurring replication of themes related to the trauma. Family members who may have escaped the trauma are inducted into playing roles in the reenactments of the survivor's traumatic experience. Over time, they become unwilling participants in these recurring patterns, and they contribute to the process of passing along the patterns— despite their experience of personally having escaped the traumatic event. In this manner, a traumatic event can establish patterns within a family that are passed from generation to generation (i.e., from members who were not subject to the original trauma to new members who were not subject to the original trauma).

An example of a trauma theme being replicated within a family relationship is that of a woman who has been raped who becomes sexually inhibited and experiences her husband as insensitive and trying to force sex upon her. In such a situation, she is again feeling like a victim and experiences her husband as the perpetrator. In his frustration, her husband may behave insensitively and come to enact the role of the perpetrator.

Sometimes the victim becomes the victimizer within the family and causes other family members to feel like the victim. For example, if members of one generation were traumatized by attacks based on their religious beliefs, they may replicate the experience with their children— perhaps by taking an equally extreme position that demands unquestioning allegiance to the beliefs. The children then may have a similar experience of helplessness and persecution related to their beliefs.

These examples of trauma replications both involve transference figures related to the trauma. In these two cases, the traumas were human-induced and the transferences involved the roles of victim and victimizer. Other roles that are often replicated include bystander, indifferent support figure, positive support figure, etc. However, trauma replications do not always involve transference relationships. The replication often centers on the expectation of a recurrence of the event, whether it was human-induced or not. For example, a survivor of a natural disaster, such as an earthquake, may react to environmental events that serve as reminder stimuli as though the earthquake is happening again. Family members, particularly the less differentiated family members, can become as sensitized to these reminder stimuli as the survivor. Similarly, someone who experienced a traumatic loss may respond to every minor separation as a new traumatic loss and, again, less differentiated family members may come to share the survivor's fear of loss/separation.

The therapist's role in regard to replications is to help the family recognize that the identified patterns are replications and to interrupt the projections that generally accompany them. This is particularly important with the less differentiated family members, as they are the most vulnerable to identifying with the projections. Whether projections are involved or not, family members fall into playing roles in the replications and, as with the caretaker children, their personalities can easily come to be confused with the roles they play in the family.

Safety Concerns

A continued concern with safety is a hallmark characteristic of a traumatized family. It is usually expressed in the family's world view in the form of suspicious, distrustful attributions concerning the motivations of others, but it can also be seen in various symptoms of family members (i.e., fearfulness, phobias, and other anxiety reactions). Family members will deal with fear differently according to the particular rules and myths of the family. For example, families that deny the experience of fear often produce counter-phobic children who get themselves into dangerous situations because of their inability to recognize fearful feelings and use them to engage in appropriately cautious behavior. On the other hand, families that are ruled by excessive fear can produce exceptionally timid children who are vulnerable to becoming dysfunctional in demanding situations.

The concern with safety is obvious in the family ruled by fear, but it is also a factor in the family that denies fear. In such families, the message being communicated is that it is not safe to feel fear, perhaps implying that fear is a disabling influence in dealing with threatening situations. Krystal (1988) notes how the signal content of the fear affect provides individuals with extremely important information in situations involving external danger. Failure to identify and experience one's own fearful feelings prevents an individual from having access to that vital information.

Therapists working with traumatized families deal with safety issues from the first moment of the therapy. The therapy setting itself must be safe before any therapeutic progress can occur. As treatment progresses, issues surface that stem from the family's particular approach to safety and the experience of fear.

Survivor Missions

A unique aspect of traumatized families is the sense of special demand and purpose that is bestowed upon the children. Every child in the family grows up with an awareness that the family has been hurt in some way, and the child must contend with the implications for his or her own identity and sense of security as well as for the survival of the family. Some children learn to deal with the family hurt by devoting their own lives to the purpose of doing something about it.

Herman (1992) has identified the survivor mission that becomes an organizing principle for the lives of many survivors and Danieli (1985) has observed the missions of the offspring of survivors. Many children of trauma survivors report feeling a certain purpose to their lives. They must achieve to justify the many sacrifices, or they must suffer in order to connect with their parents and give meaning to the incomprehensible pain. They must struggle with the same demons or they must champion the same cause. One way or another, the child's life choices are strongly influenced by the mission he or she adopts.

Sometimes, in their rush to ensure that they are not susceptible to the same terrors, many offspring of traumatized families inadvertently inflict new terrors through their distorted and constricted relations with their own children. For example, they may fail to nurture the child when he or she hurts and instead require the child to be invulnerable. A common result is that the child is then unable to bring his or her sensitive side into connections with others and thus becomes an insensitive person.

It should be noted that many survivors have found the pursuit of a mission to be an adaptive means of coping with some major trauma in the life of the family. Pursuing a mission can give life meaning and purpose, qualities that are often extinguished (perhaps not destroyed) in severe traumatization.

Symptomatic Members

The presence of symptomatic members provides an ongoing source of traumatic stress in the family. As noted above, members having reexperiencing symptoms can induce non-traumatized members into playing a role in reenactments of the trauma. But even without being pulled into reenactments, other family members are highly stressed by having to contend with a loved one who is continually being traumatized by his or her reexperiencing symptoms. Members with avoidance symptoms exert a powerful influence on the family's freedom and daily life. Avoidance symptoms frequently play a role in the development of safety issues among less differentiated members. Symptomatic members who are perpetually numb increase the level of insensitivity within the family.

Perhaps the most difficult symptom for other family members is when one individual lives in a state of hyperarousal. Whether expressed through irritability, rage attacks, or sleep problems, hyperarousal problems are very difficult to live with—both for the symptomatic member and for those who must accommodate the symptomatic member's symptoms. Additionally, many individuals with hyperarousal develop secondary problems—such as alcoholism or workaholism—that create further turmoil for the rest of the family. Whatever the nature of the affected member's symptoms, living with such an individual can constitute an extreme stressor for the entire family.

The therapist's role with symptomatic members is to see that the affected individual receives specific help, such as in the form of medication and/or adjunctive therapy, as well as to help the family identify the need to structure family life realistically. This can be a delicate area because the therapist must avoid the trap of making the symptomatic member too much of an "identified patient" and thereby turn the family problem into an individual problem.

CHANGING THE BURNOUT ENVIRONMENT

When a therapist has the opportunity to help a traumatized family, the first level of intervention occurs when the therapist establishes a new kind of relationship with the family. The therapy often occurs in a relational space that the family has never visited before, one that operates according to different rules. In the therapy hour, every family member's needs, feelings, and point of view are regarded as legitimate and important. Listening carefully, working at understanding and accepting others' feelings—these become the rules that govern the therapist–family system.

The rules of the therapy and their non-judgmental but firm enforcement by the therapist provide a sense of security, a necessary ingredient for the traumatized. Security in therapy can refer to physical safety, such as learning to maintain an optimal physical distance, pacing, and predictability with some physically insecure clients. However, more often, security in therapy is related to the relational trauma more than the primary or physical trauma. The survivor is excruciatingly sensitive to being blamed or shamed for his or her actions. The therapist directs family members to communicate more openly, in a non-shaming, non-attacking manner. Members are not allowed to speak for others, to gang up on someone, or to discount others' feelings.

The result of the expressive rules and emotionally and physically secure environment of therapy is an atmosphere where traumatic affect can be surfaced, discussed, and processed, both emotionally and cognitively.

The Therapy Process

The initial focus of family therapy is determined by the family's symptoms, problems, and complaints when they enter therapy. If these problems relate to a failure to process the primary trauma, then processing the primary trauma becomes an early meta-goal (i.e., a larger goal to be sought even while responding to the more immediate demands of daily complaints). In addition, the relational trauma may require processing if the family has suffered severe relational breaks.

Since the goal of family therapy is always to resolve the presenting problem, processing the primary and relational traumas is mandated only if the family can see the relevance of resolving those issues in order to resolve the presenting problem (Catherall, 1988). Thus, an early goal of the therapy is to ensure that the family understands that processing issues related to the trauma is necessary to achieve resolution of the presenting problem. While processing, the therapist must stay attuned to the ways in which the family interrupts the process. These interruptions frequently represent reactions to violations of the maladaptive rules.

It is also helpful to take a strong stand on the family's reliance on ineffective coping strategies. The existence of ineffective strategies may be easily explained in terms of family of origin patterns, but their continued deleterious influence must not be ignored. The therapist needs to help the family articulate and hold onto their desire to live by more adaptive strategies in the present. Changing a lifetime of ineffective coping behaviors is not easy; the family needs encouragement, hope, and patience from the therapist.

The Mechanisms at Work

The following examples illustrate some of the dynamics of traumatized families. The first is a family with a traumatized parent, the second is an example of transgenerational effects of traumatization, and the third is a couple dealing with an ongoing source of traumatic stress.

Example 1: The K Family

Mr. K was severely traumatized as a result of his combat experience in Vietnam. His reaction to the experience was likely compounded by his childhood experience of being passed around among various relatives, all of whom showed little interest in taking care of him. Mrs. K grew up in an alcoholic family in which she assumed responsibility for taking care of her younger siblings and also for her mother whenever the mother was incapacitated by drinking. When Mr. K's reexperiencing symptoms became very pronounced, he lost his job; he alternately went for long periods without leaving the house and at other times would leave and disappear for days at a time. He had severe sleep problems and often would work himself into a state of exhaustion in order to sleep. When he was without work, he sometimes would exhaust himself through physical exercise.

Mr. and Mrs. K had two children, an early-adolescent son and a preadolescent daughter. The boy actively defended his father when others became upset with the father's irresponsible behavior. The girl found ways of fleeing the environment through involvement at school and with friends. When the father was home, he often sat in front of the TV and was uncommunicative. No one in the family challenged this behavior. The mother worked to maintain the family and was always busy, apparently too busy to give the kids sufficient attention. The father worked inconsistently after losing his job; whenever he worked, he did so to such an intense level that several times he burned himself out. Usually, this was after an initial period of greatly impressing his newest employer.

Mr. and Mrs. K presented with problems related to Mr. K's continued reexperiencing and hyperarousal symptoms and Mrs. K's concern about how to provide the best environment for Mr. K in the home. As therapy progressed, the problems changed to include the unexpressed conflict between them and eventually included the children's anger and disappointment with their father. Throughout the therapy, Mr. K worked on his primary trauma at the VA. The couple came for the first several sessions, then the children joined the therapy and came for several sessions, interspersed with couples sessions.

Many dynamics of traumatized families were apparent in this case. It was helpful early in the therapy to identify and discuss Mrs. K's caretaker history. Though she was aware of it, she had not really discussed it with anyone, and she was less aware of the ways in which it continued to be manifested in her current life. As she examined her tendency to assume a caretaker role (because of her experience in an alcoholic family of origin), she began to relinquish some of the less helpful aspects of the role and to take better care of herself, an activity she previously regarded as selfish. She took more responsibility for meeting her own needs, along with refusing to meet as many of her husband's needs as she had been meeting. The result was that she became less angry with her husband.

As the therapy progressed, the entire family came to treat the father as less fragile; even the children began to express their disappointment and anger with him. Mr. K initially became very depressed and angry with this change. He experienced the family as not caring about him, similar to the relatives with whom he had been placed as a child. However, he was helped to express these concerns and the family responded. Though he still struggled with feeling unloved, he couldn't help but see that his family was standing by him. The myth that father was fragile and the associated rule that father must not be confronted each slowly changed. The most difficult point was when the son quit defending the father and expressed his own anger at him for the periodic disappearances.

Throughout the family therapy, the father continued to work on the primary trauma. When he experienced the family as less supportive, his symptoms intensified. As he worked through the family's changed relationship with him, his symptoms became less intense. Perhaps the most important change for him was his acquisition of more effective coping strategies. He quit running away from the family when he was most distressed. He became more able to express his feelings at those times and consequently felt increasingly connected, even when he was feeling beleaguered by his symptoms.

At the point at which therapy stopped, some dysfunctional rules and coping strategies had changed. The son more freely expressed his anger at his father, but in doing so he was still able to remain connected. The member of the family who had changed the least was the daughter. She continued to utilize her father's strategy of disconnection and she remained cut off from the rest of the family. The mother made several positive changes in her own life and felt much more comfortable with herself. The father was less symptomatic and had learned to maintain a better connection with the family even when he was going through a period of distress. Perhaps most importantly, all the family members were more authentic and present with each other, although the daughter still lagged behind the others.

Example 2: The T Family

Both Mr. and Mrs. T had trauma in their families of origin. Mr. T was the adult child of two Holocaust survivors. He was born in Europe and moved to the United States at an early age. Mrs. T was the child of a broken family. She was the only one of the children in the family who bore a strong resemblance to the father, and this contributed to her being a frequent target of her mother's anger. Mr. and Mrs. T had a number of ongoing conflicts, but the usual theme was Mrs. T's complaint that Mr. T worked incessantly and was emotionally inaccessible and Mr. T's complaint that Mrs. T constantly criticized him and dumped her anger on him.

Mr. and Mrs. T entered therapy to deal with their marital conflict and Mrs. T's reported depression. For a while, the therapy focused on resolving the daily conflicts that dominated their relational life. As therapy progressed, exploration into family-of-origin issues began to reveal the depth of the trauma in their backgrounds. They began to see themselves less as victims of one another and more as the heirs of the many traumatic sequelae that persisted in their families of origin. As their relationship improved, each showed increased empathy for the other. The meaning of Mr. T's emotional constriction and Mrs. T's feelings of persecution and abandonment changed. They were not so much doing these things to each other as struggling to have a relationship despite the relational injuries of the past.

As their self-understanding and their understanding of each other improved, many traumatic sequelae became clear. Mr. T's workaholic pace came to be understood in terms of his parentified role in his family of origin and his mission in life—to live a life that made up for the family's suffering. He was the child in his family who assumed responsibility for the management of resources. He became the primary breadwinner as a teenager. He recalled having to take such adult responsibilities as buying cars, negotiating loans, and dickering with creditors because his parents did not speak English. He assumed considerable responsibility for his mother's emotional health; he was the only one who could deal with her when she became profoundly demoralized and dysfunctional. Additionally, the family environment was alexithymic—there was little recognition of feelings. No one was attuned to his emotional needs or able to help him learn to negotiate the fulfillment of those needs within relationships.

Mrs. T was understanding about the emotional constriction of Mr. T's family background and became more patient in her efforts to tune into him and, in so doing, facilitate his tuning into himself. Also, both Mr. and Mrs. T gained a better understanding of Mrs. T's feelings of abandonment and her quickness to resort to hostility. As Mr. T came to take Mrs. T's irritable, critical behavior less personally, she became more vulnerable and revealed how much she needed his support. She was so accustomed to being the family black sheep that she had learned to hide her vulnerable feelings and needs behind a caustic, demanding facade. She came to see how much her mother had projected the blame for the breakup of the family onto her. Over the years, she learned to live up to the role of the problem child, while simultaneously fighting and denying the guilt and blame that were directed at her. The result was that she learned to beat others to the punch at blaming.

Mr. T gradually came to identify some specific myths that existed in his family of origin. No one in the family ever revealed weakness or vulnerability, except when the mother would fall apart (but even then she remained paranoid and denied her vulnerability). Several of the extended family members had survived labor camps during the Holocaust, an environment where those who appeared weak were transported to death camps. Thus, the family myth was that showing weakness would lead to destruction. Mr. T had learned to deal with his mother's breakdowns in a mechanical, controlled manner. The family's belief/myth was that mother would decompensate even further if she received an empathic response that encouraged the emotionality. Consequently, Mr. T became even more unemotional and controlled when Mrs. T became upset. That response only fueled Mrs. T's distress at those times.

Mr. and Mrs. T remained in therapy for several years, off and on, and eventually achieved a stable connection. A recent contact confirmed that they have maintained a warm, expressive, mutually supportive relationship.

Example 3: The M Family

Mr. and Mrs. M had a quiet, childless marriage. They seldom conflicted and they shared many interests. Neither was very social, but they agreed about the few friendships that they maintained. Life went well for them; Mr. M was very successful financially, and Mrs. M was happy to maintain the home. However, after several years together, Mr. M developed a major, chronic disease. In the initial phase, his life was at great risk. After that, he was stabilized but continued to require extensive treatment. Their lifestyle naturally came to revolve around his treatment and they made many lifestyle changes. Mrs. M was very supportive throughout. However, after several years, Mrs. M developed a major depression.

Both Mr. and Mrs. M used a stoic style of coping, denying a personal need for support but trying to be there for each other. Since Mr. M's illness placed his physical needs on center stage, Mrs. M devoted herself to helping him achieve the adjustments in his lifestyle that his chronic condition demanded. They did not talk about their mutual fears and Mrs. M kept her feelings of increasing isolation and hopelessness to herself. They were around each other a great deal yet they came to feel more distant. Mr. M's personal management style changed at work; he became considerably more sensitive and thoughtful in his dealings with his staff. However, he was unable to transfer his more sensitive style of relating to his relationship with Mrs. M. He did not know how to reach her, and when her symptoms of depression became severe, he desperately sought professional help.

Mr. and Mrs. M entered conjoint therapy and began to learn how to communicate more fully with each other. As therapy developed, they also began to learn how their early life experiences had contributed to their difficulties with connecting. Mr. M was the youngest of eight siblings. The family was extremely non-communicative; Mr. M did not learn that some of his siblings were from an earlier marriage until he was grown. When Mr. M was seven years old, his father was disabled in an accident. No one focused on Mr. M's feelings and needs; he was left to deal with the devastation to the family on his own. He responded by becoming exceptionally independent, a condition that brought him many worldly successes but few relationships.

When Mr. M was 18 years old, he fell in love with a girl who was killed in an accident. He became depressed and dysfunctional for a period but eventually recovered. When Mrs. M became depressed, he saw her laying on the couch in a fetal position that reminded him of his girlfriend who had died. That was when he realized the depth of her depression and became motivated to seek help. Just as the death of the girlfriend seemed to revive the empty, hopeless feelings that Mr. M was not free to express when his father was disabled, the sight of Mrs. M's depressed state again stirred Mr. M's desperate fear of losing his loved one.

Mrs. M grew up in another constricted family environment. Her father was a bitter, caustic man who felt exploited by his family of origin. When he was teenager, he was unable to prevent a brother from bleeding to death. Later, when he returned from World War II, he was forced to exhaust all his resources taking care of his mother and felt his siblings did not do enough to help. In his marriage to Mrs. M's mother, he was verbally abusive, and Mrs. M became the family peacemaker and her mother's emotional caretaker. Thus, Mrs. M's own feelings and needs went unexpressed. To this day, she resists sharing her problems with anyone from her family of origin for fear of again being disappointed.

Mr. and Mrs. M's experience is an example of how growing up in a disconnected, unexpressive environment ill prepares people to deal with major stressors. Mr. M fell back on the independent, self-care style that he learned as a boy. He wanted to connect with Mrs. M, but he lacked the skills that he might have learned in a more expressive family.

Mrs. M resumed her selfless, caretaking role and did not know how to express her own feelings and needs in the midst of her concern for her husband. These non-expressive communication styles, unmet needs, and premature levels of responsibility were Mr. and Mrs. M's legacies from growing up in burned-out family environments.

CONCLUSION: THE SELF OF THE THERAPIST

In the cases presented, as in all work with traumatized families, the self of the therapist plays a key role in the first level of intervention (i.e., in creating a new kind of environment in the therapy sessions). The therapist must be personally authentic and connected. The relationship with the family must be mutually empathic, which means that the family must feel that they have an impact upon the therapist at the same time that the therapist is influencing them. The therapist has to maintain a therapeutic alliance that respects the needs, feelings, and point of view of all the family members and not simply those who have the power or those who are symptomatic (Pinsof & Catherall, 1986). By truly listening to every family member and treating every member's point of view as legitimate, the therapist lays the foundation for a new mode of connecting that makes it possible to change those mechanisms that have maintained the burnout environment.

REFERENCES

Bowen, M. (1966). The use of family theory in clinical practice. *Comprehensive Psychiatry, 7,* 345–374.

Catherall, D.R. (1988). Interviewing in family therapy: The problem centered approach. In E. Lipchik (Ed.), *Interviewing* (pp. 49–69). Rockville, MD: Aspen Publishers.

Danieli, Y. (1985) The treatment and prevention of long-term effects and intergenerational transmission of victimization: A lesson from Holocaust survivors and their children. In C.R. Figley (Ed.) Trauma and Its Wake: The Study and Treatment of Post-Traumatic Stress Disorder, New York: Brunner/Mazel, 295–313.

Donovan, D.M., & McIntyre, D. (1990). *Healing the hurt child: A developmental-contextual approach.* New York: W.W. Norton & Co.

Feldman, L.B., & Pinsof, W.M. (1982). Problem maintenance in family systems: An integrative model. *Journal of Marital and Family Therapy, 8,* 295–308.

Figley, C.R. (1988). A five-phase treatment of family traumatic stress. *Journal of Traumatic Stress, 1*(1), 127–141.

Figley, C.R. (1989). *Helping traumatized families*. San Francisco: Jossey-Bass.

Figley, C.R. (1995). *Compassion fatigue: Coping with secondary traumatic stress in those who treat the traumatized*. New York: Brunner/Mazel.

Figley, C.R., & McCubbin, H.I. (Eds.) (1983). *Stress and the family, Volume 2: Coping with catastrophe*. New York: Brunner/Mazel.

Herman, J.L. (1992). *Trauma and Recovery*. U.S.A.: Basic Books.

Jackson, D.D. (1957). The question of family homeostasis. *The Psychiatric Quarterly Supplement, 31,* 79–90.

Jordan, J.V. (1989). Relational development: Therapeutic implications of empathy and shame. *Work in progress, No. 23*. Wellesley, MA: Stone Center Working Paper Series.

Jordan, J.V. (1991a). The meaning of mutuality. In J.V. Jordan, A.G. Kaplan, J.B. Miller, I.P. Stiver, and J.L. Surrey (Eds.), *Women's growth in connection: Writings from the Stone Center* (pp. 81–96). New York: The Guilford Press.

Jordan, J.V. (1991b). Empathy, mutuality, and therapeutic change: Clinical implication of a relational model. In J.V. Jordan, A.G. Kaplan, J.B. Miller, I.P. Stiver, and J.L. Surrey (Eds), *Women's growth in connection: Writings from the Stone Center* (pp. 283–289). New York: The Guilford Press.

Jordan, J.V., Kaplan, A.G., Miller, J.B., Stiver, I.P., & Surrey, J.L. (1991). *Women's growth in connection: Writings from the Stone Center*. New York: The Guilford Press.

Kramer, J.R. (1985). *Family interfaces: Transgenerational patterns*. New York: Brunner/Mazel.

Krystal, H. (1988). *Integration & self-healing: Affect, trauma, alexithymia*. Hillsdale, NJ: The Analytic Press.

Maruyama, M. (1963). The second cybernetics: Deviation-amplifying mutual causal processes. *American Scientist, 51,* 164–179.

McCubbin, H.I., & Figley, C.R. (1983). Bridging normative and catastrophic family stress. In H.I. McCubbin and C.R. Figley (Eds.), *Stress and the family, Volume 1: Coping with normative transitions* (pp. 218–228). New York: Brunner/Mazel.

Miller, J.B., & Stiver, I.P. (1991). A relational reframing of therapy. *Work in progress,* Wellesley, MA: Stone Center Working Paper Series.

Minuchin, S. (1982). Reflections on boundaries. *American Journal of Orthopsychiatry, 52,* 655–663.

Pinsof, W.M. (1995). *Integrative problem-centered therapy: A synthesis of family, individual, and biological therapies*. New York: Basic Books.

Pinsof, W.M., & Catherall, D.R. (1986). The integrative psychotherapy alliance: Family, couple, and individual therapy scales. *Journal of Marital and Family Therapy, 12*(2), 137–151.

Stiver, I.P. (1990a). Dysfunctional families and wounded relationships—Part I. *Work in progress,* Wellesley, MA: Stone Center Working Paper Series.

Stiver, I.P. (1990b). Dysfunctional families and wounded relationships—Part II. *Work in progress,* Wellesley, MA: Stone Center Working Paper Series.

Stiver, I.P. (1991). The meaning of care: Reframing treatment models. In J.V. Jordan, A.G. Kaplan, J.B. Miller, I.P. Stiver, and J.L. Surrey (Eds.), *Women's growth in connection: Writings from the Stone Center* (pp. 250–267). New York: The Guilford Press.

Wilson, J.P. (1989). *Trauma, transformation, and healing: An integrative approach to theory, research, and post-traumatic therapy.* New York: Brunner/Mazel.

INDEX